Robert H Garman, DVM

Wolfe Veterinary Series

Further titles now in preparation:
A Colour Atlas of Veterinary Dermatology
A Colour Atlas of Veterinary Ophthalmology
A Systemic Pathology of Domestic Animals

A COLOUR ATLAS OF NEOPLASIA IN THE CAT, DOG AND HORSE

A Colour Atlas of

Neoplasia in the cat, dog and horse

D.E. Bostock
MA, Vet MB, MRCVS
Lecturer in Animal Pathology
Department of Clinical Veterinary Medicine
University of Cambridge

L.N. Owen
MA, DVSc, FRCVS
Assistant Director of Research
Department of Clinical Veterinary Medicine
University of Cambridge

Wolfe Medical Publications Ltd
10 Earlham Street, London WC2

Year Book Medical Publishers, Inc.
35 East Wacker Drive, Chicago, Ill. U.S.A.

Studentlitteratur
Lund, Sweden

Published by Wolfe Medical Publications Ltd, 1975
Printed by Smeets-Weert, Holland
SBN 7234 0633 2

Distributed in Continental North, South and Central America,
Hawaii, Puerto Rico, and the Philippines by
Year Book Medical Publishers, Inc
By arrangement with Wolfe Medical Publications Ltd
Printed by Smeets-Weert, Holland
Library of Congress Catalog Card Number: 75-18538
International Standard Book Number: 0-8151-1079-0

Acknowledgements

We should like to thank Professor W I B Beveridge for help and advice. Dr A R Jennings has contributed considerably to our efforts and we are very grateful to him. Many of the tumours illustrated have been used in aetiological and therapeutic studies and we wish to thank the Cancer Research Campaign and the Medical Research Council for their support.

Illustrating this Atlas would have been impossible without the help and kindness of many friends and colleagues who have most generously allowed publication of photographs from their collections. We would particularly like to thank Mr B Bagnall, Dr W S Bailey, Dr K C Barnett, Mr W R Cook, Mr S W Douglas, Dr T Hanichen, Col J Hickman, Dr O Jarrett, Dr D F Kelly. Mr R B Lavelle, Mr M C G Littlewort, Dr J McHowell, Mr P A Neal, Dr A C Palmer, Mr T Turner, Mr R G Walker and Mr H D Williamson.

We should also like to thank Mr H E Bowman, Mr K Hunt, Mr P Lancaster and Mrs J Patten for technical assistance.

The classification of tumours in this Atlas is that used by the World Health Organisation.

Table of Contents

Introduction

With the increased use of vaccines and antibiotics in domestic animals death due to infectious disease has decreased dramatically in the last two decades. Consequently neoplasia has become of greater importance to the practising veterinarian and more of his time is now employed in the diagnosis, prognosis and treatment of tumours.

Until recently our knowledge of the biological behaviour of even the commonly occurring animal tumours was scanty, and many surgically excised neoplasms were not subjected to histological examination. However, with the increasing sophistication of veterinary practices and the laboratory services provided for them this position is rapidly being rectified.

As well as forming an important part of veterinary practice the animal neoplasms provide an excellent model for the study of cancer in man. They approach the human situation very closely in that they arise spontaneously in an outbred population which, in the case of the dog and cat, shares a similar environment to man.

BENIGN AND MALIGNANT NEOPLASMS

A neoplasm may be defined as a multiplying collection of cells which are not under the control of the homeostatic mechanisms of the body. Tumours are divided into benign and malignant types, the following criteria being amongst the most important for their differentiation:

	Benign	**Malignant**
Structure	Typical of the particular tissue of origin.	Often atypical, differentiation imperfect.
Mode of growth	Usually purely expansive with encapsulation. Invasion of vessels and spaces rare.	Infiltrative as well as expansive so that encapsulation is absent. Invasion of vessels common.
Rate of growth	Usually slow. Nuclear chromatin normal. Nucleoli normal.	May be slow or rapid. Often many mitotic figures. Chromatin hyperchromatic. Nucleoli large.
Metastasis	Absent.	Frequently present.
Recurrence after removal	Rare.	Frequent.
Stroma	Abundant.	Usually scanty.
Cell size and morphology	Uniform.	Pleomorphic.
Significance to the host	Dangerous because of: (a) Position, or (b) Accidental complications, or (c) Production of excess of hormone.	Intrinsically dangerous because of progressive infiltrative growth or metastasis.

CLASSIFICATION

Tumours are classified according to their tissue of origin. All malignant tumours arising from tissue of mesodermal origin are *sarcomas*, the actual tissue of origin being indicated by a prefix. Thus *lymphosarcoma* is by definition a malignant tumour of lymphoid tissue and *rhabdomyosarcoma* a malignant tumour of striated muscle.

Malignant ecto- and endo-dermal tumours are *carcinomas,* the prefix *'adeno'* indicating that they are derived from glandular tissue. Again the tissue of origin is indicated by a prefix so that a sebaceous gland adenocarcinoma is a malignant tumour of sebaceous cells, while a squamous cell carcinoma is a non-secretory tumour of prickle cells.

Benign mesenchymal tumours are classified by the name of the tissue of origin followed by '*oma*' thus the benign counterparts of the tumours previously mentioned would be *lymphoma* and *rhabdomyoma.* The nomenclature of benign ecto- and endo-dermal tumours is not, however, so straightforward. Benign tumours of secretory cells are termed *adenomas*, further classified by a prefix (*e.g. sebaceous adenoma, adrenal cortical adenoma*) while benign non-secretory tumours are designated *papillomas.* A basal cell tumour is an exception to the general rule since it is a benign tumour which may look malignant. *Melanoma* is a tumour with a benign name which may be benign or malignant.

BIOPSY AND SUBMISSION OF SPECIMENS TO LABORATORIES

A special biopsy punch can be used but generally a scalpel is perfectly adequate. It is important to ensure that the biopsy specimen includes the underlying tumour and is not merely overlying normal, necrotic, or inflammatory tissue. Thus a thin sliver of tissue which extends deeply into the mass is much better than a rectangular portion from the more superficial layers. Wherever possible a biopsy should include the junction between normal and abnormal tissue. If the entire tumour is excised it may be fixed in 10% formol saline or other suitable fixative intact provided it is not more than 1cm in diameter, but if it is larger a representative portion only should be fixed. This should have an area of 1–2cm^2, a thickness of not more than 5mm and necrotic tissue should be avoided wherever possible. In general the volume of fixative should be at least 10 times that of the tissue to be fixed.

If these general rules are observed the tissue can be despatched by post immediately after removal and will be fixed and ready for further processing on arrival at the laboratory. Special forms are usually available from laboratories and these should be correctly completed and sent with the tumour. Prognosis is intimately connected not only with the histological appearance of the tumour but with many other factors including the age of the animal and the site and size of the tumour. The pathologist should thus have as much information as possible.

TREATMENT OF NEOPLASMS

Some Principles of Surgical Treatment

- *Examine the animal for systemic disturbances such as anaemia, renal and heart disease or pyometra, and for metastatic lesions, particularly in the regional lymph nodes and lungs, before surgical excision of a primary tumour is attempted.*
- *Excise a generous quantity of normal tissue around the tumour at the time of operation and avoid cutting into the tumour itself. If this is done accidentally discard the scalpel as contaminated and carry on with a fresh blade. It is very easy to transfer tumour cells via the blade, especially with sarcoids in horses and feline mammary carcinomas.*
- *Excise the draining lymph nodes where suspect, particularly the inguinal nodes in posterior mammary tumours in the bitch. If there is no palpable evidence of metastasis, it is probably better to leave the nodes in situ.*
- *Submit the excised tumour for histological examination.*
- *Check for tumour recurrence or metastasis at frequent intervals.*

Radiotherapy

- *Always have a histological diagnosis and choose only those tumours which are likely to respond to X-irradiation. Tumours showing a good response include anal adenomas, carpal 'granulomas', reticulum cell tumours, mastocytomas, the transmissible venereal tumour, some squamous cell carcinomas and some melanomas.*
- *In valuable horses consider the use of radioactive gold implants. Give the radiotherapist the site and dimensions of the tumour so that the dose and distribution of the gold grains can be determined.*
- *Radiotherapy is of most value when used prophylactically to prevent recurrence following surgical excision. Ideally the site should be irradiated immediately following surgery or after 10 days have elapsed. If employed from 2–6 days post-operatively the wound may never heal.*

Chemotherapy

- *Chemotherapy is only palliative.*
- *Facilities must be available for haematological examination during therapy, as many of the drugs used depress the bone marrow.*
- *Whenever possible work in collaboration with a member of the staff of a veterinary or human hospital who has a good knowledge of the subject.*

Hormonal Therapy

- *Stilboestrol or hexoestrol implants produce temporary regression of anal adenomas and corticosteroids are of palliative value in canine lymphoid tumours.*

Chapter 1
The Skin and Adnexa

Because of the accessible nature of the site, tumours of the skin and subcutaneous tissues are generally presented at an earlier stage than those in other organs and in most practices provide about 45 % of all tumour-like masses presented for surgical excision. Common benign skin neoplasms include basal cell tumours, papillomas and trichoepitheliomas from the epidermis, and fibromas, lipomas and haemangiopericytomas from the connective tissue elements of the dermis. In addition, the glandular tissues of the adnexa may undergo neoplastic transformation to produce adenomas of sweat, sebaceous, and hepatoid glands, whilst there are a variety of other cells situated in the dermis which can give rise to benign tumours, including melanoblasts, mast cells, reticulum cells and histiocytes.

Up to 20 % of lesions removed from the skin, and believed initially to be neoplastic, prove to be of a non-neoplastic nature on histological examination, the commonest type of lesion in this category being the granuloma. Other non-neoplastic conditions which can be mistaken for tumours include various cysts, especially the epidermal cyst encountered so commonly in the dog, calcinosis circumscripta, haematomas, and abscesses.

About 40 % of the total number of true tumours removed from the skin and adnexa prove to be malignant. These include the malignant counterparts of the benign tumours mentioned earlier, lymphosarcomas and secondary tumours from malignancies elsewhere. Skin metastases are very rare in all the domestic animals, but occasionally secondary spread from mammary and other carcinomas is seen in the dog and cat.

EPITHELIAL TUMOURS OF THE SKIN AND ADNEXA

Papillomas

Occurrence and gross appearance

In the horse multiple small tumours occur in young adults, mainly around the lips and nostrils (*1*), whilst larger solitary lesions are seen in older animals.

In the dog and cat papillomas are unusual but may be found occasionally, mainly in old animals. They are generally less than 0.5cm in diameter and can occur anywhere on the body, although the eyelids, face and limbs are most commonly affected. The gross appearance of the tumours is similar in all three species, lesions consisting of numerous small horny projections arising from a broad, flat base (*2*).

Histological appearance

The dermal connective tissues are hyperplastic, and thrown up into finger-like projections covered by numerous layers of well differentiated prickle cells, with obvious keratinisation of the superficial layers. The rete pegs are elongated and branching, but there is no evidence of invasion of the connective tissues by isolated cell nests (*3*).

Aetiology

The aetiology of these tumours in old animals is unknown. Multiple papillomas in young adult horses are caused by a host-specific papova virus.

Treatment and prognosis

Many papillomas in the dog and cat are not treated unless they become ulcerated and bleed, when surgical removal results in a complete cure. The viral papillomas of horses will regress spontaneously, but this can take up to two years. Regression may occur in some cases following vaccination using a minced suspension of some of the lesions treated with 0.1% formalin. Four subcutaneous injections of 5–10ml at weekly intervals is the usual procedure. Claims have been made that intramuscular injections of Lithium Antimony Tartrate are of value.

Papillomatous proliferation of the skin of the ear in white cats and the penile epithelium of old horses is a precancerous change and should be treated as such, by radical excision.

Squamous Cell Carcinomas

Occurrence and gross appearance

Squamous cell carcinoma, the malignant counterpart of the papilloma, is derived from the prickle cells of the epidermis which penetrate the stratum germinativum and invade the underlying connective tissues. This tumour is relatively common in all three species and occurs in the external nares, eyelids, ears (*4*) and skin of the lips in cats, especially in those animals where these areas are not pigmented; in the eyelids, skin of the penis, and vulval lips in old horses; and in the external nares and skin of the limbs, flanks and back in dogs.

In cats, the cutaneous squamous cell carcinoma is usually a fairly small, very erosive lesion, with a raised firm edge, which can be confused with an eosinophilic granuloma (*see page 111*) when it occurs on the external nares or lips. Its cut surface is whitish in colour and very firm in consistency.

In the dog and horse squamous cell carcinomas are proliferative rather than crateriform and appear as ulcerated, fungating lesions with a poorly defined border (**5** *and* **6**).

Histological appearance

Squamous cell carcinomas consist of a dense fibrous stroma, which is frequently heavily infiltrated by inflammatory cells, and which separates irregular foci of malignant prickle cells. Individual tumours vary considerably in their degree of histological maturity and grading of the tumours into histological types is relatively simple (*7 and* **8**). Follow-up studies have suggested that these grades are of prognostic significance in the cat, and probably in other species.

Aetiology

The aetiology of this condition is unknown, but it has been suggested that smegma may be carcinogenic, resulting in penile carcinomas in horses, whilst the propensity for white cats to develop the tumour on the ear tips and other exposed sites has been ascribed to the effects of sunlight. A precancerous lesion known as photo-allergic dermatitis, which may exist for several years before true neoplasia develops, is well documented in the cat.

Treatment and prognosis

Treatment is by radical surgery. In the horse, where the tumours are usually well differentiated, amputation of the entire penis, vulval lips, or eyelid may result in a cure, although poorly differentiated tumours metastasise to the regional lymph nodes. Radioactive gold implants are of value in the treatment of incompletely operable tumours, for example those of the eyelid and skin of the orbit.

In the cat, surgery must be extremely radical wherever possible if local recurrence is to be avoided, and should include removal of the regional lymph nodes. Most cats with well differentiated tumours will be cured by radical excision, but where the tumour is poorly differentiated local recurrence and metastasis are likely; the survival time in these cases generally being less than six months from the first operation.

Squamous cell carcinomas in the skin of dogs are usually well differentiated and small tumours can be cured by surgical excision. The unusual, poorly differentiated tumours behave in a similar manner to those in the cat and should be treated in the same way.

In both dogs and cats, surgery followed by fractionated X-irradiation to a total dose of 4,000R is of value in those cases where it is suspected that excision was incomplete.

1

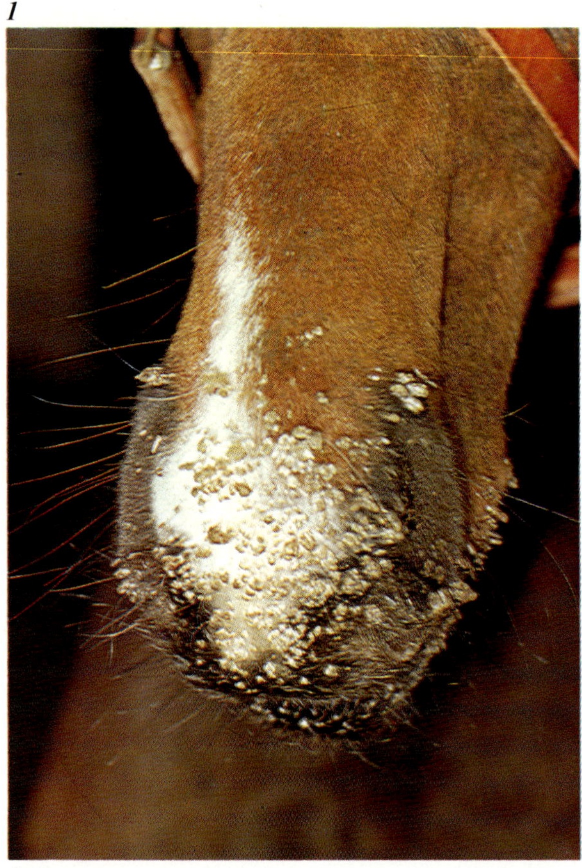

2

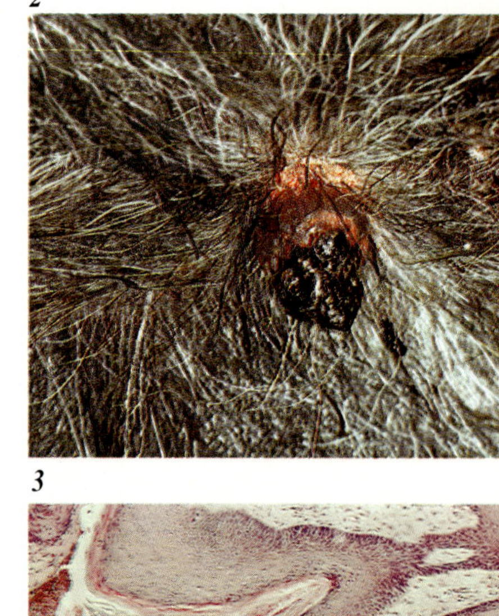

3

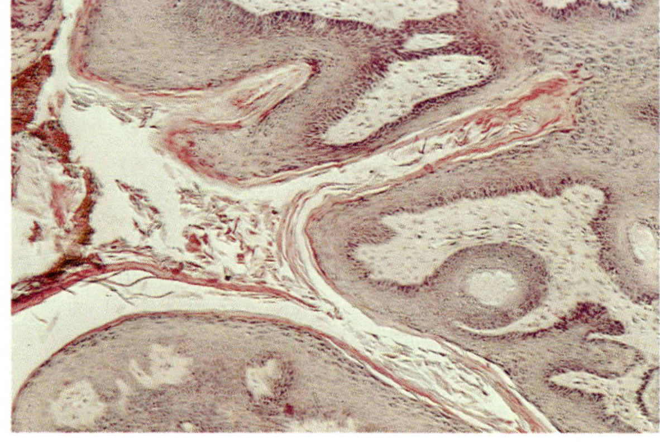

4

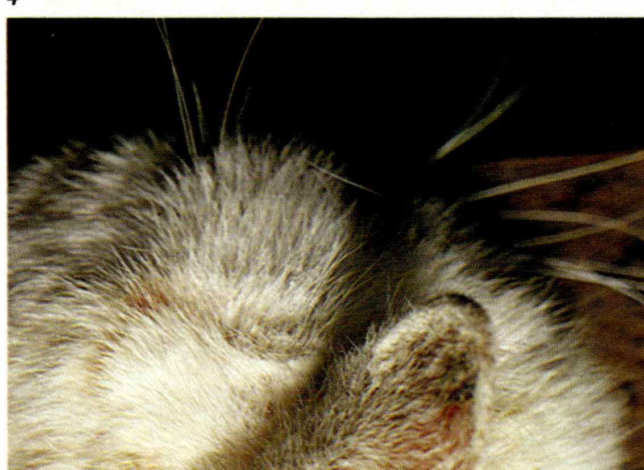

1 *Multiple viral papillomas around lips and nostrils of a two-year-old horse.*

2 *Papillomas in skin of head. 11-year-old Miniature Poodle.*

3 *Papilloma – horse. H & E.*

4 *Early squamous cell carcinoma of pinna in an old white cat. Note the erosive nature of the lesion.*

5 *Squamous cell carcinoma of the vulva in a 23-year-old mare.*

6 *Squamous cell carcinoma of the penis in a gelding.*

7 *Well differentiated squamous cell carcinoma showing central 'pearls' of mature keratin – dog. H & E.*

8 *Poorly differentiated squamous cell carcinoma in which keratinisation is minimal – cat. H & E.*

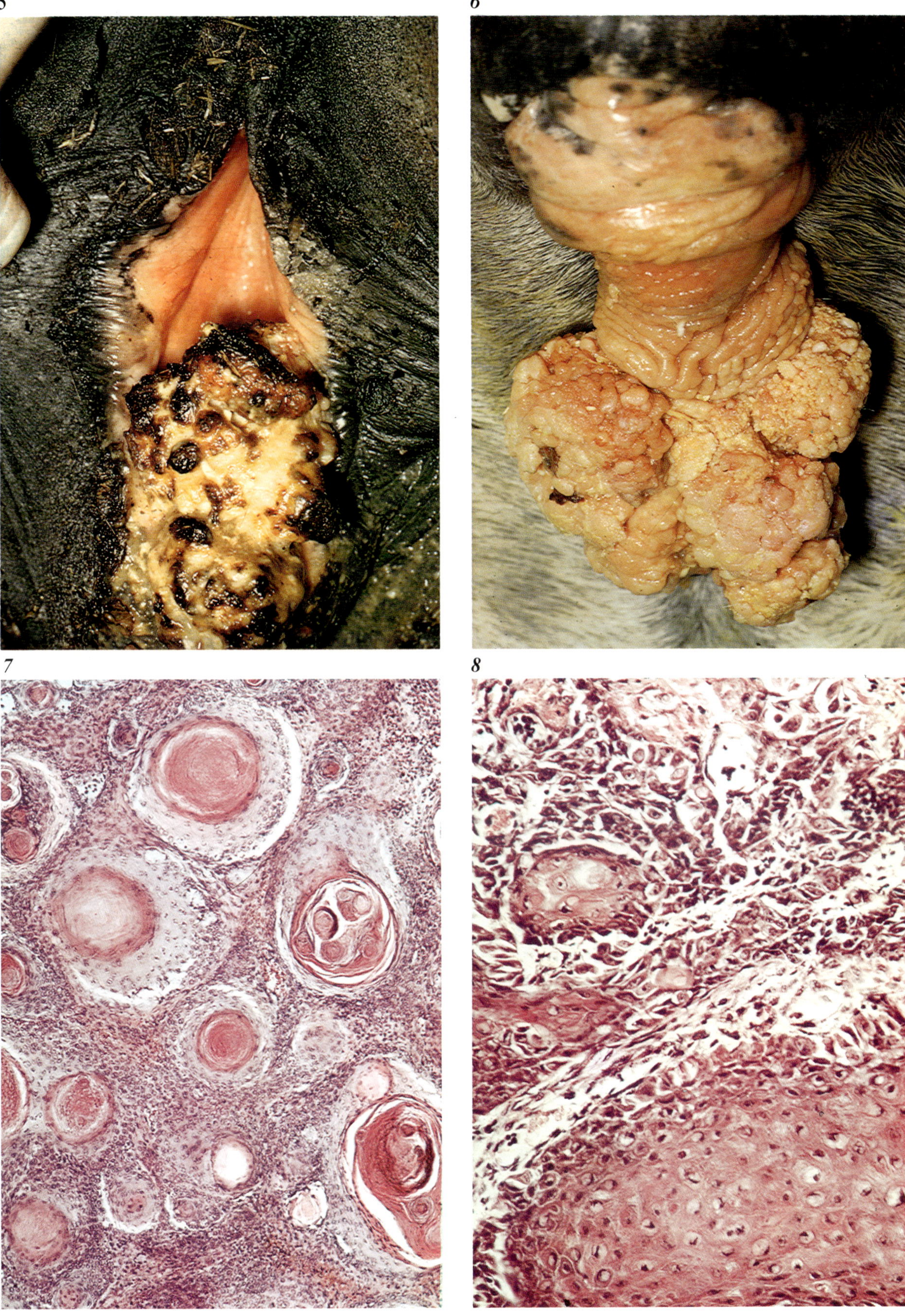

5
6
7
8

Basal Cell Tumours

Occurrence and gross appearance

These tumours occur frequently in dogs, particularly in Spaniels, where they nearly always appear in the skin of the face or limbs (***9***). They are also found fairly commonly in cats but are less common in horses. The lesions are proliferative rather than ulcerative and the gross appearance is of a roughly oval, well circumscribed mass, firmly attached to the epidermis, but mobile over the underlying tissues. They grow slowly but can become very large, ulcerate through the skin and become secondarily infected.

In dogs and cats basal cell tumours may be intensely pigmented due to melanin pigment in the cells, when they can be confused with melanomas on gross examination (***10***).

Histological appearance

The microscopic appearance is variable, although the different forms have no prognostic significance. The most common type of tumour is well circumscribed but not encapsulated, and consists of an abundant fibrous stroma which contains large, brick-shaped, hyperchromatic cells arranged as characteristic festoons or chains, but never forming closed acinar structures (***11***). Other forms consist of solid foci of cells separated by a fibrous stroma with the outermost layer of cells being palisaded, with the long axis of the cells arranged radially (***12***). Occasionally, and especially in the cat, a few cells towards the centre of the focus can become keratinised, this type being termed a baso-squamous tumour (***13***). In the dog, basal cell tumours which are forming hair follicle-like structures, with a central, clearly defined zone of mature keratin, are termed trichoepitheliomas (***14***).

Treatment and prognosis

Surgical excision of even the larger tumours is relatively simple, since they are confined to the skin, and results in a complete cure. Following adequate surgery local recurrence and metastasis are rare.

Sebaceous Gland Tumours

Occurrence and gross appearance

Benign tumours of the sebaceous glands are very rare in the horse and cat, but common in old dogs where they appear most frequently as small, firm, smooth and pedunculated nodules, often affecting the eyelids (***15***), although other areas of the skin can be involved. These lesions, which rarely grow above 0.5cm in diameter, are often called 'warts' (***16***) and may be multiple. Occasionally, larger sebaceous adenomas occur and these can be found anywhere in the skin. They are firmly attached to the epidermis, which tends to ulcerate and become infected, but are mobile over the underlying tissues. True carcinomas are rare and are impossible to distinguish from large adenomas grossly.

Histological appearance

There is considerable variation in the histological appearance of these tumours. They may be composed of small, solid lobules of discrete, well differentiated, fat filled cells (***17***), or a closely packed sheet of smaller, very hyperchromatic, reserve cells, only a few of which are showing evidence of sebaceous differentiation (***18***). Squamous metaplasia is sometimes conspicuous. These tumours do not exhibit encapsulation and the distinction between adenomas composed mainly of reserve cells, and true carcinomas is often very fine. Carcinomas have less tendency towards sebaceous differentiation and contain more mitotic figures however (***19***).

Treatment and prognosis

Surgical removal of even histologically malignant tumours will usually result in a cure. A small proportion of carcinomas recur locally, and will, rarely, produce metastases in regional lymph nodes or lungs.

9 *Basal cell tumour in the forelimb of a seven-year-old dog.*

10 *Heavily pigmented multiple basal cell tumours in a Chihuahua.*

11 *Basal cell tumour with 'Medusa Head' appearance. H & E.*

12 *Solid basal cell tumour. Note the palisaded appearance of the outermost zone of cells. H & E.*

13 *Baso squamous tumour – cat. H & E.*

14 *Trichoepithelioma – dog. The cells are forming discrete hair follicle-like structures. H & E.*

15 *Sebaceous adenoma in lower eyelid of a dog.*

16 *Sebaceous adenomas, skin of the head in a 12-year-old dog.*

17 *Sebaceous adenoma composed of small lobules of well defined, fat filled cells. H & E.*

18 *Sebaceous adenoma with closely packed reserve cells. Squamous metaplasia is apparent in some areas. H & E.*

19 *Sebaceous gland adenocarcinoma. Only a few cells show evidence of sebaceous differentiation. H & E.*

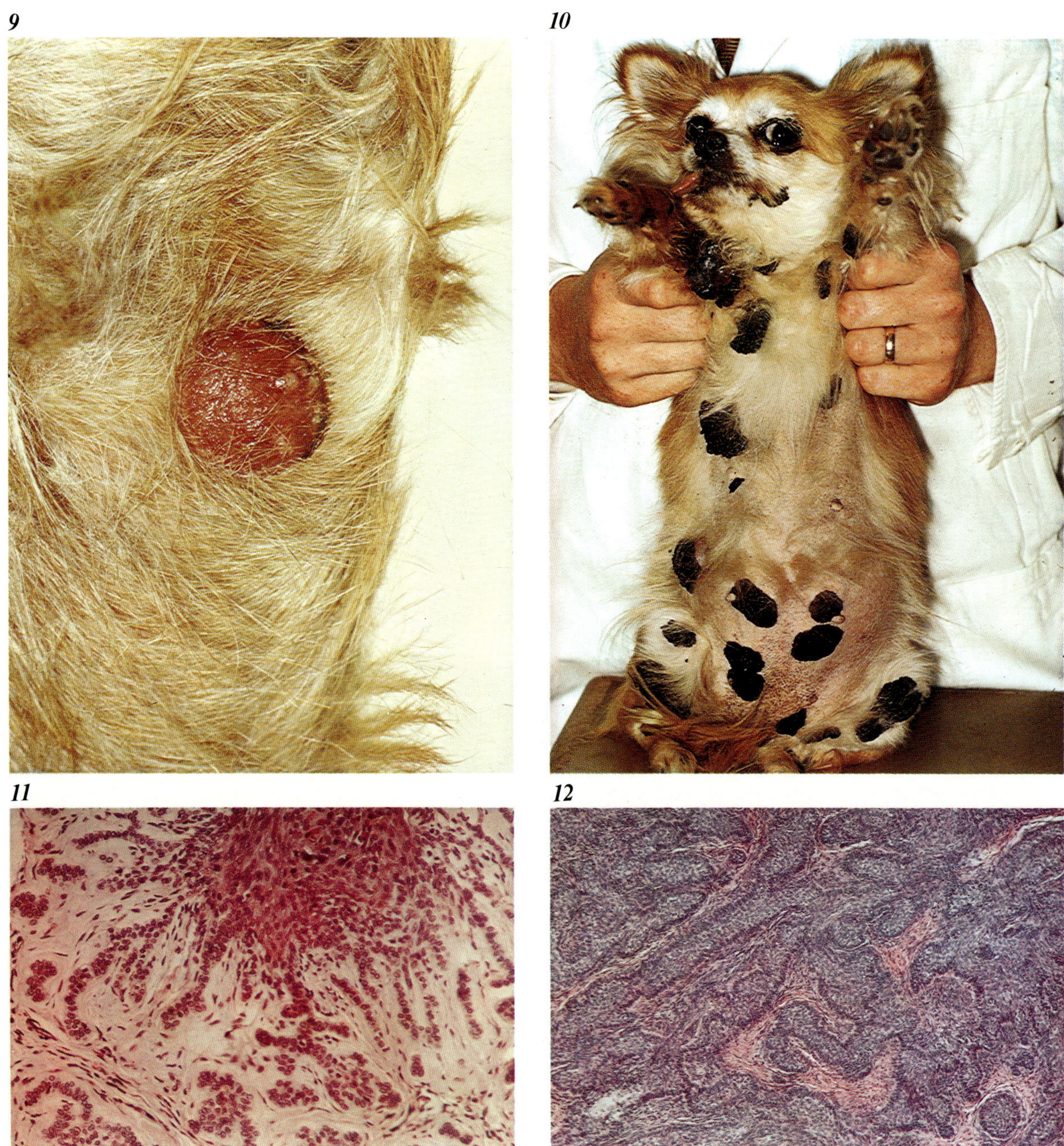

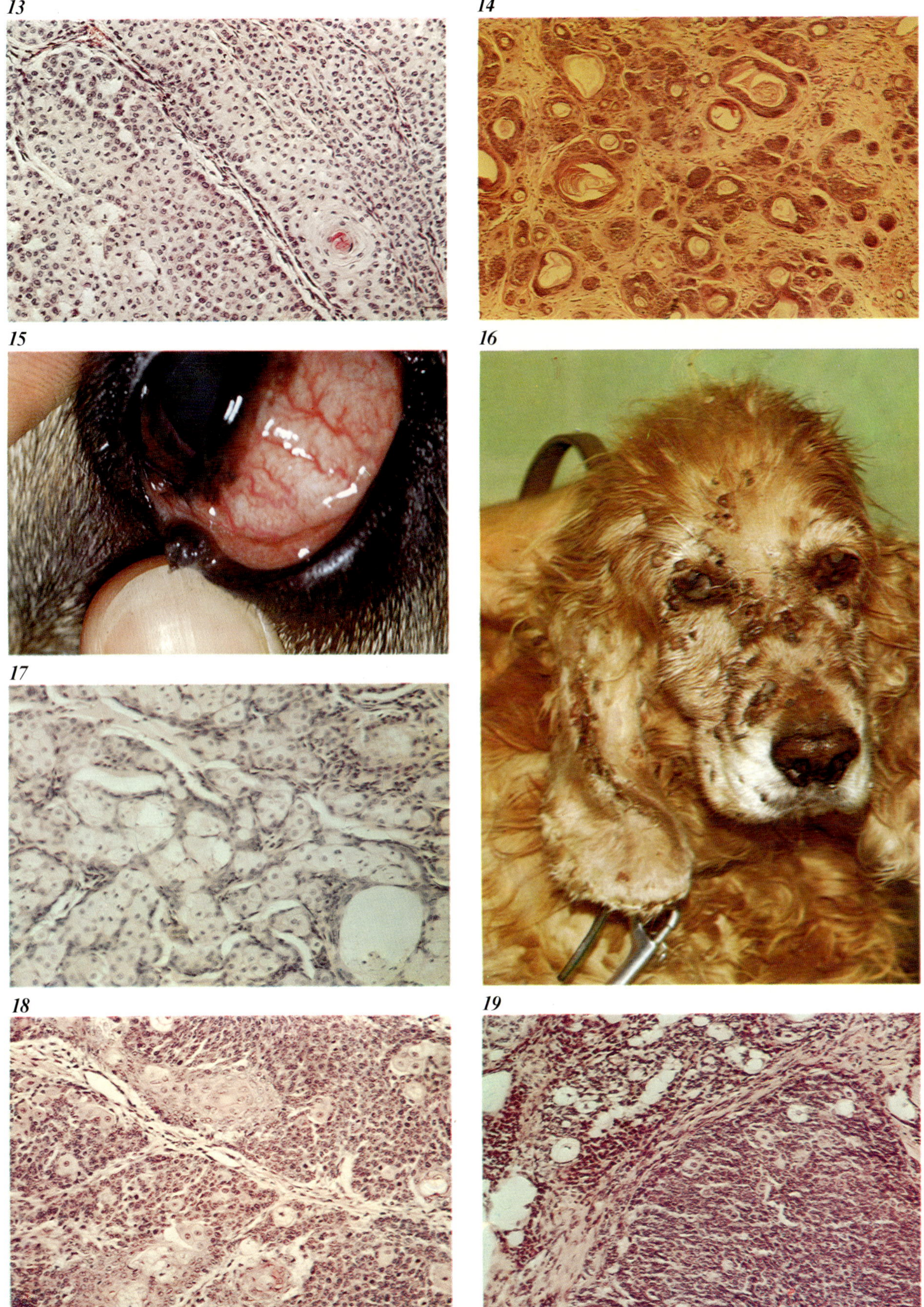
13
14
15
16
17
18
19

Hepatoid Gland (Perianal) Tumours

Occurrence and gross appearance

These tumours are derived from secretory cells which are very similar to sebaceous cells and which occur only in the dog. They are found particularly around the anal ring and also occur on the dorsal and ventral surfaces of the base of the tail and in the skin lateral to the prepuce. Tumours are common in old male dogs, but more unusual in females. They often appear as multiple, small, firm nodules beneath the skin, although a single large tumour can sometimes be seen. They eventually ulcerate (***20***) and in some advanced cases cause difficulty in defaecation. They have a rubbery texture and a pinkish cut surface which can be seen to be divided into numerous tiny lobules.

Histological appearance

Benign tumours are much commoner than carcinomas and appear histologically as numerous, well circumscribed solid foci of large, clearly defined epithelial cells with a central spherical nucleus and abundant eosinophilic cytoplasm (***21***). Squamous metaplasia is often a marked feature, but is not of prognostic significance.

Carcinomas of hepatoid glands are not common, but are distinguished histologically by the more poorly differentiated nature of the cells, which are closely packed and have a basophilic nucleus and scanty cytoplasm (***22***). Mitotic figures are common and vascular invasion may be obvious.

Aetiology

Some tumours are under hormonal control but the exact aetiology is obscure.

Treatment and prognosis

Surgical removal can be difficult owing to the size and site of the tumour, and about 35% of adenomas around the anal ring recur following surgical excision. Many large tumours can be reduced in size before surgery by castration. The administration of stilboestrol or hexoestrol implants (*15–30mg subcutaneously*) will also lead to tumour regression but this is usually of a temporary nature.

These tumours are radiosensitive and fractionated doses to a total of 3,000R X-irradiation frequently result in long term regression. Anal adenocarcinomas usually recur locally after removal and may metastasise to the iliac lymph nodes or lungs.

Ceruminous Gland Tumours

Occurrence and gross appearance

These tumours arise in the ceruminous glands of the external auditory meatus and are found only in the dog and cat, where they are the commonest intra-auricular neoplasm. They are relatively more common in cats than dogs, and occur in the deeper parts of the external canal where they may initially be diagnosed as otitis externa. They are usually less than 1cm in diameter, well circumscribed, pinkish in colour and dome shaped. Ulceration and superficial secondary infection are common.

Histological appearance

Even the well differentiated tumours are not encapsulated and show evidence of local infiltration. They consist of more or less regular acinar or papillary structures, lined by one or more layers of columnar cells and contain a hyaline secretion (*23*). The more malignant tumours are less well differentiated and show marked invasion of the stroma, sometimes with vascular infiltration.

Treatment and prognosis

The prognosis should be guarded as benign tumours tend to recur after surgical excision and metastasis to the parotid lymph node may occur from carcinomas (*24*). Forms of treatment other than surgery are of little value.

20 *Ulcerated hepatoid adenoma – eight-year-old male Alsatian (German Shepherd).*

21 *Hepatoid adenoma. The tumour consists of clearly defined lobules of large epithelial cells.*

22 *Hepatoid adenocarcinoma. This section is from a lung metastasis.*

23 *Ceruminous gland adenoma – dog. H & E.*

24 *Adenocarcinoma of ceruminous gland. This tumour recurred after surgery and metastasised to the parotid lymph node.*

20

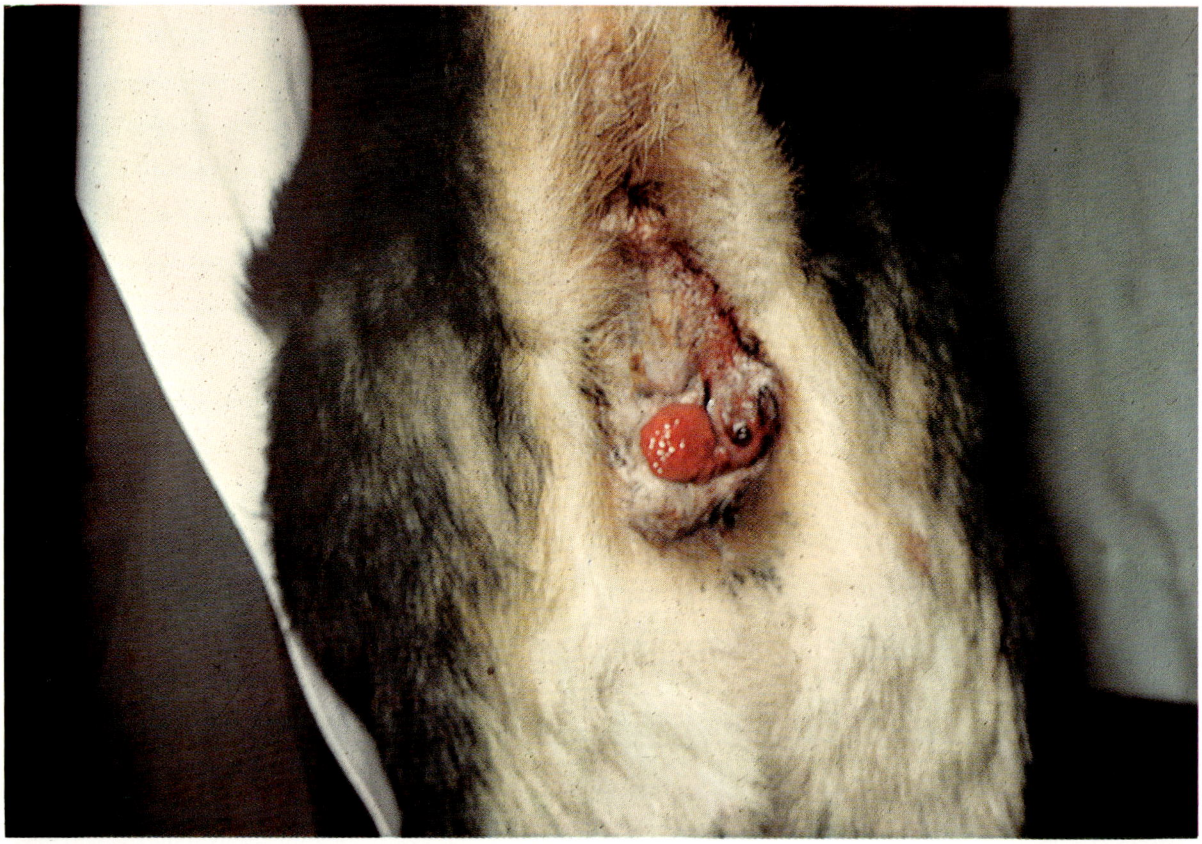

21 **22**

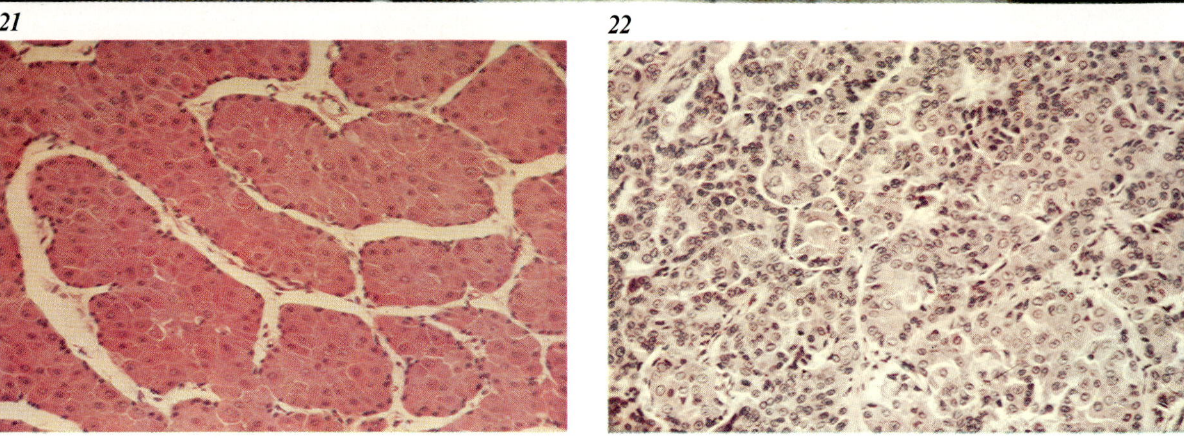

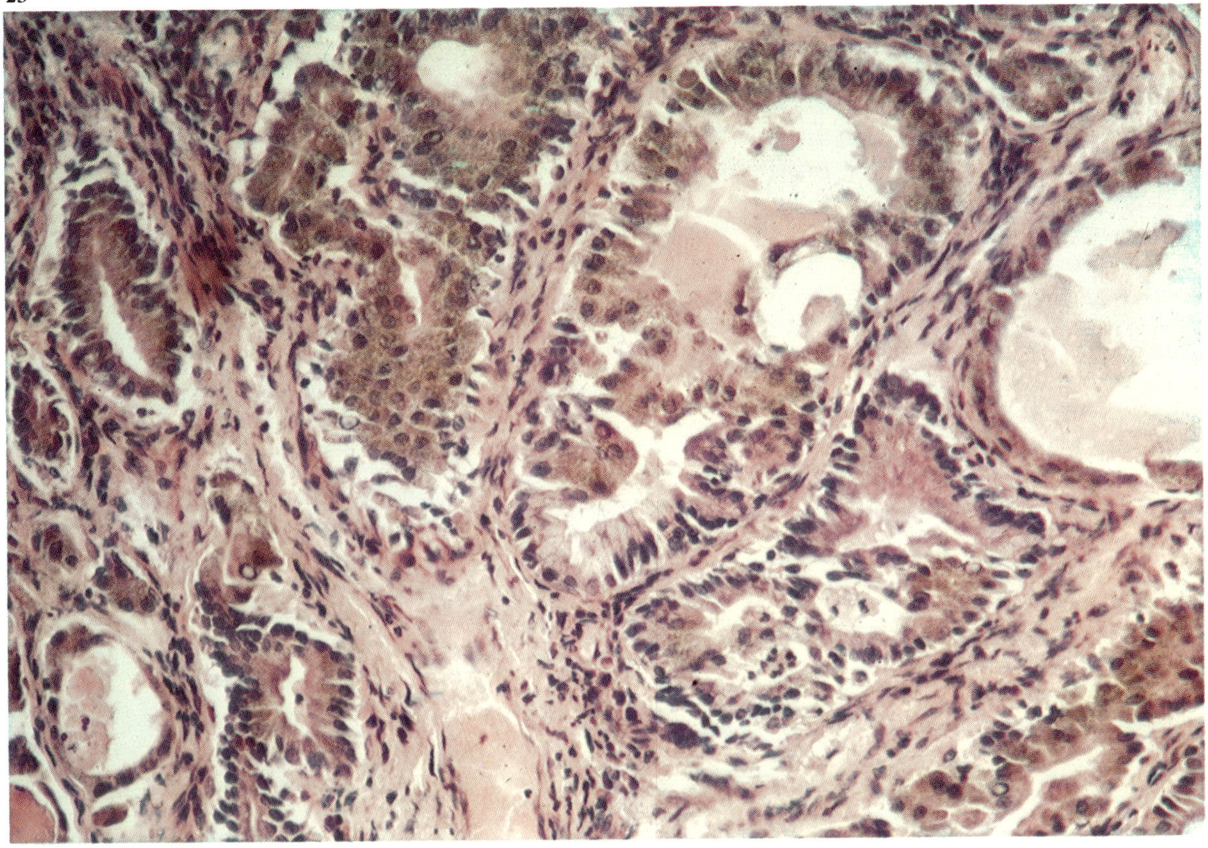

24

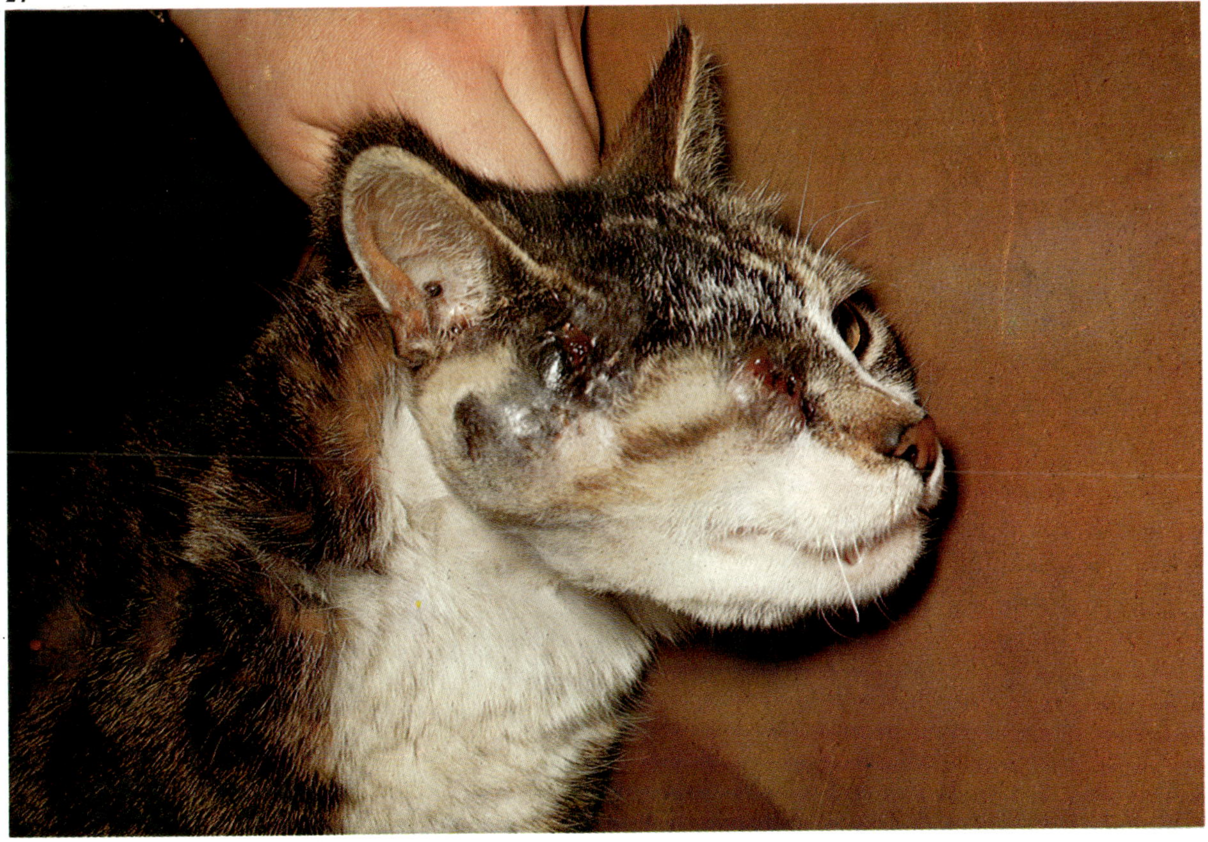

Sweat Gland Tumours

Occurrence and gross appearance

These tumours are uncommon in the dog and rare in the other species. In dogs they usually arise in the subcutaneous tissues of the back, flanks, or legs, and appear as firm, well circumscribed masses which are closely attached to the overlying skin, but which do not normally ulcerate. They are usually 1–2cm in diameter, but can become much larger. The cut surface may be white and homogeneous, or may contain small cysts filled with a clear, yellowish fluid (***25***).

Histological appearance

Encapsulation is not seen and the likelihood of malignancy must be judged from the degree of differentiation. Benign tumours consist of a fibrous stroma separating well defined acinar or cystic structures lined by a single layer of cuboidal cells often thrown up into branched papillary ingrowths (***26***). The lumen of the acinus contains a hyaline secretion in some cases.

Sweat gland carcinomas are less well differentiated. They tend to be papillary, although solid and tubular forms also occur (***27***). Rarely, benign and malignant mixed tumours may arise from sweat glands in dogs.

Treatment and prognosis

Even in histologically malignant sweat gland tumours local recurrence and metastasis are unusual following surgical excision. The prognosis should thus be favourable in all cases except those in which there is obvious vascular invasion on histological examination.

Melanomas

Occurrence and gross appearance

Skin melanomas are of most importance in the dog, are also fairly common in the horse, but are very uncommon in cats. They are seen most frequently in old grey or dappled horses, where they are often multiple and tend to occur especially around the preputial opening, the vulva, the anus, and on the abdomen (***28***). They are usually fairly small, measuring from 0.5–3cm in diameter, well circumscribed, firm, dome shaped, and have an intensely pigmented cut surface (***29***). Occasionally tumours may be much larger. They are closely adherent to the skin and ulceration is usual in the more advanced case.

In the dog, melanomas fall into two distinct categories. Older dogs may develop multiple, darkly pigmented nodules, usually from 0.5–1cm in diameter in the skin of the lower abdomen (***30***), limbs, or head. These lesions are rubbery in consistency, often pedunculated, well circumscribed, superficial, and grow very slowly.

The other type of melanoma in this species is usually solitary, occurs especially on the limbs or tail (***31***), and is firm and locally invasive. This type of tumour may grow rapidly and ulcerate through the overlying skin. Canine melanomas are rarely as darkly pigmented as those in the horse and some tumours are amelanotic, either completely or in part.

Melanomas in cats are unusual, but those seen have been single, superficial and well circumscribed masses which grow up to several centimetres in diameter.

Histological appearance

These tumours are never encapsulated, although the more benign ones are well circumscribed, and consist of large, closely packed, polygonal cells, with a spherical or oval, hyperchromatic nucleus, a moderate amount of basophilic cytoplasm and very indistinct cell boundaries. Sometimes the cells are spindle shaped and arranged in whorls or parallel bundles, but do not produce an obvious intercellular matrix. In all save the most poorly differentiated tumours some cells will contain intracytoplasmic melanin granules (***32***) which may be so numerous as to obscure the cytoplasm entirely.

Aetiology

This is unknown but it has been stated that every grey horse, if it lives long enough, will develop melanomas.

Treatment and prognosis

Melanomas in the horse grow relatively slowly but regional lymph node and visceral metastases are common (***29***), so that, especially where tumours are numerous, the prognosis must be guarded. Surgical excision is the only treatment which has been used extensively and cures are possible when all the nodules can be removed at an early stage.

In the dog the small multiple type of tumour is benign, and carries a favourable prognosis even when present in large numbers. The solitary, invasive tumours are malignant and can metastasise to the regional lymph nodes and lungs, although this generally occurs relatively late in the course of the disease. The main problem with this type of tumour is local recurrence, which should be expected following surgical excision. Radical excision of the tumour by amputation of the tail or limb is sometimes possible but if amputation is not feasible surgical excision followed by fractionated X-irradiation up to a total of 3,000–4,000R can produce useful remissions.

25 *Sweat gland cyst adenoma from the back of a 10-year-old dog. H & E.*

26 *Sweat gland adenoma. Note the well differentiated tubules and abundant stroma. Van Gieson.*

27 *Sweat gland adenocarcinoma – dog. H & E.*

28 *Multiple malignant melanomas in skin of prepuce – 10-year-old grey gelding.*

29 *Metastatic malignant melanoma in superficial inguinal lymph nodes – horse. The primary tumour can also be seen around the preputial opening.*

30 *Multiple benign melanomas on the ventral abdomen of an eight-year-old dog. These tumours may ulcerate and bleed.*

31 *Section of solitary melanoma in the tail of a Black Labrador. The tumour is partly amelanotic.*

32 *Malignant melanoma – dog. Note the spindle shaped cells packed with melanin granules. H & E.*

25

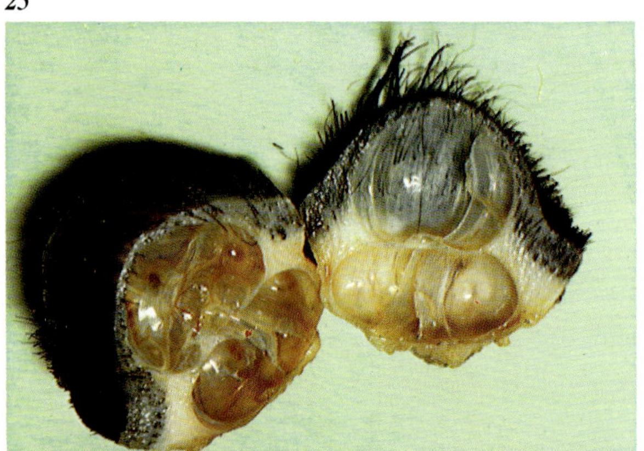

27

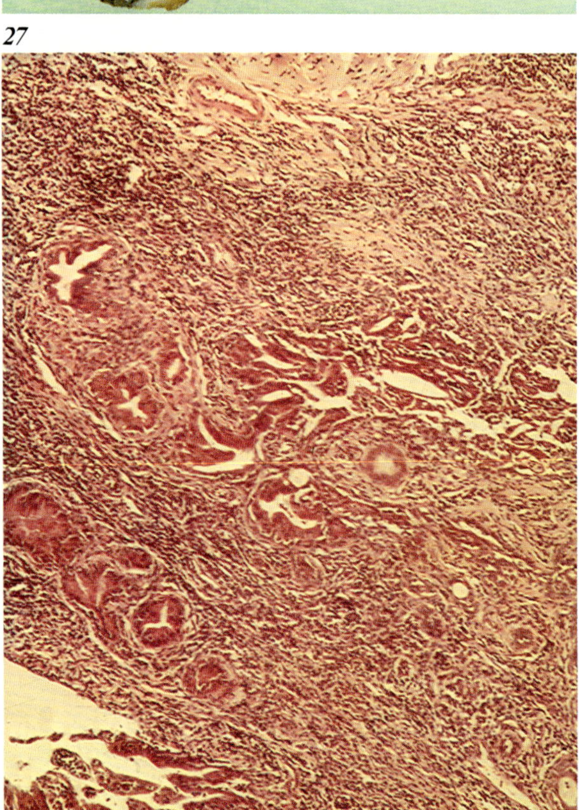

26

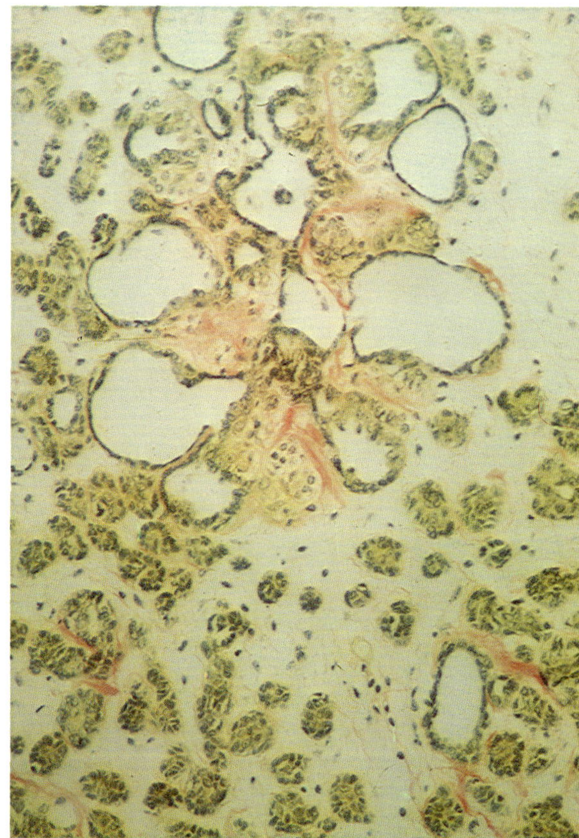

28

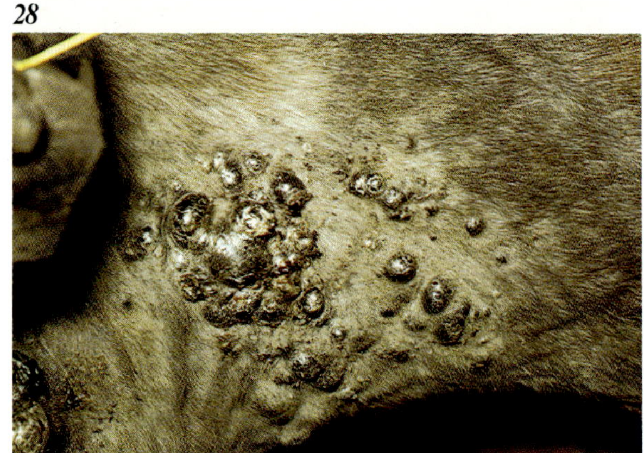

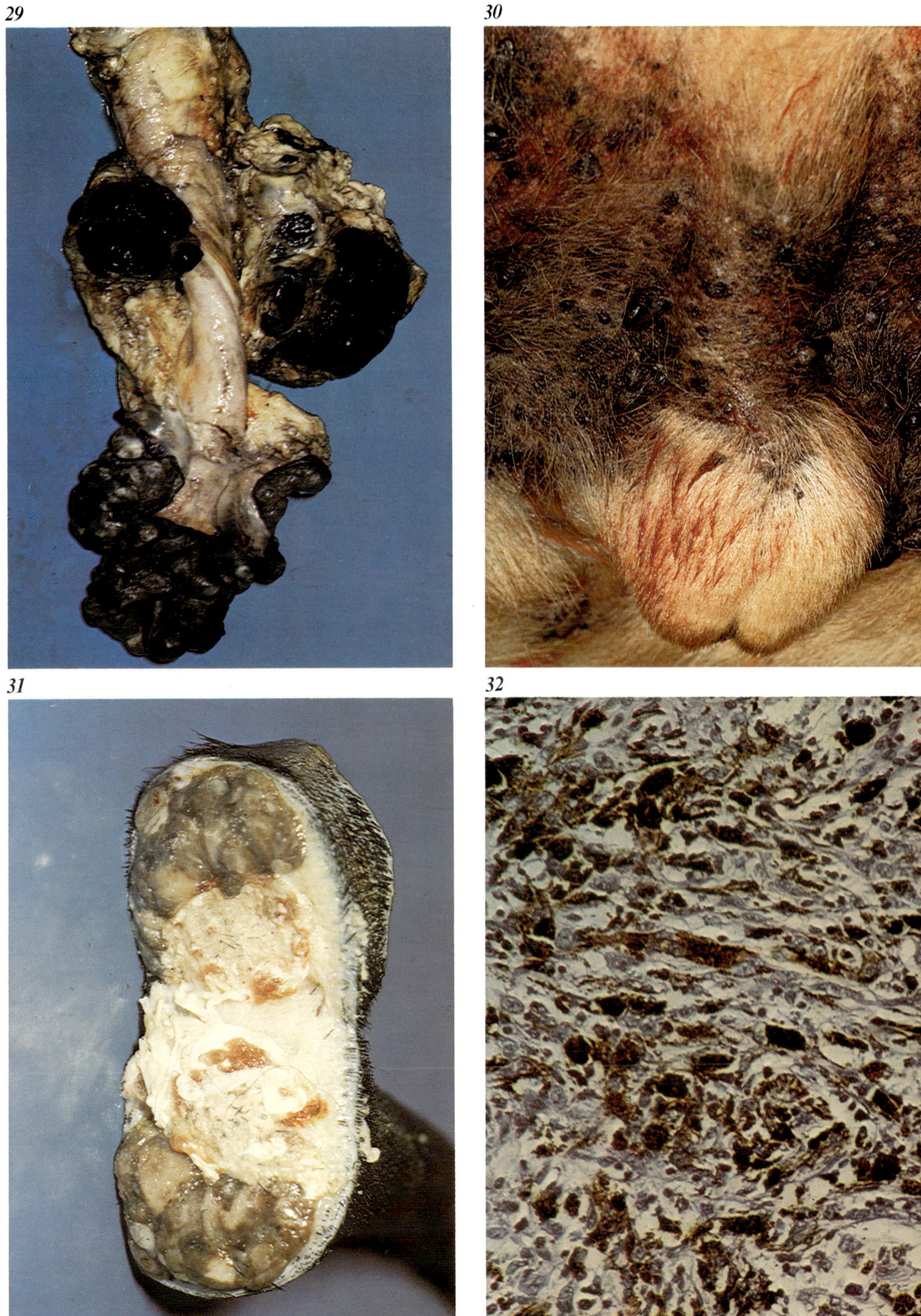
29
30
31
32

MESENCHYMAL TUMOURS OF THE DERMIS

Fibromas and Fibrosarcomas

Occurrence and gross appearance

These tumours are commonly occurring superficial neoplasms in all three species. They may occur anywhere in the skin, although, in the horse, tend to be found particularly on the face, limbs and groin.

Fibromas are well circumscribed and closely attached to the overlying epidermis which usually loses its hair (*33*). They do not readily ulcerate and are mobile over the deeper tissues. They may be firm or soft and on section have a white or yellowish, fibrous surface. Benign tumours are seen most often in the dog, less frequently in the horse and rarely in the cat.

Fibrosarcomas grow much faster, and usually attain a greater size, than fibromas. They characteristically ulcerate through the skin at an early stage in their development (*34*), are diffusely invasive, firm in consistency and firmly attached to the surrounding tissues, from which they are very difficult to remove. In the horse, fibromas and low grade fibrosarcomas tend to be multiple and are called 'equine sarcoids' (*35*).

Histological appearance

Fibromas are composed of whorls and large wavy bundles of mature collagen fibres which are produced by relatively few small, elongated cells, each with an oval, hyperchromatic nucleus (*36*). They are well defined, although not always encapsulated.

Fibrosarcomas show a marked gradation in their histological appearance from tumours which closely resemble fibromas (*37*) but with some infiltration of the surrounding tissues (*38*) to a homogeneous sheet of large, spindle-shaped cells closely packed together and arranged in a haphazard fashion. As the tumour becomes less well differentiated, the cells become larger, the nucleus less densely staining, and mitotic figures more common. The amount of intercellular collagen is progressively reduced and invasion of the surrounding tissues more obvious. In the horse, fibromas and low grade fibrosarcomas (equine sarcoids) frequently show, in addition to fibroblastic proliferation of the dermal connective tissue, acanthosis and hyperkeratosis of the overlying epidermis (*39*). This type of tumour has been termed a fibropapilloma although it is not certain whether the proliferation of the epidermis is a neoplastic or hyperplastic change.

---

33 *Fibroma in the vulva of a six-year-old Terrier.*

35 *Multiple low grade fibrosarcomas (equine sarcoids) in the inguinal region of a six-year-old horse.*

37 *Well differentiated fibrosarcoma – cat. H & E.*

39 *'Equine sarcoid'. The overlying epidermis is acanthotic and hyperkeratotic. H & E.*

34 *Fibrosarcoma in skin of forelimb – cat.*

36 *Subcutaneous fibroma – dog. H & E.*

38 *Edge of fibrosarcoma. Note the widespread invasion of surrounding muscle. Masson's trichrome.*

40 *Marsden Mark II Implantation Gun for insertion of radioactive gold seeds.*

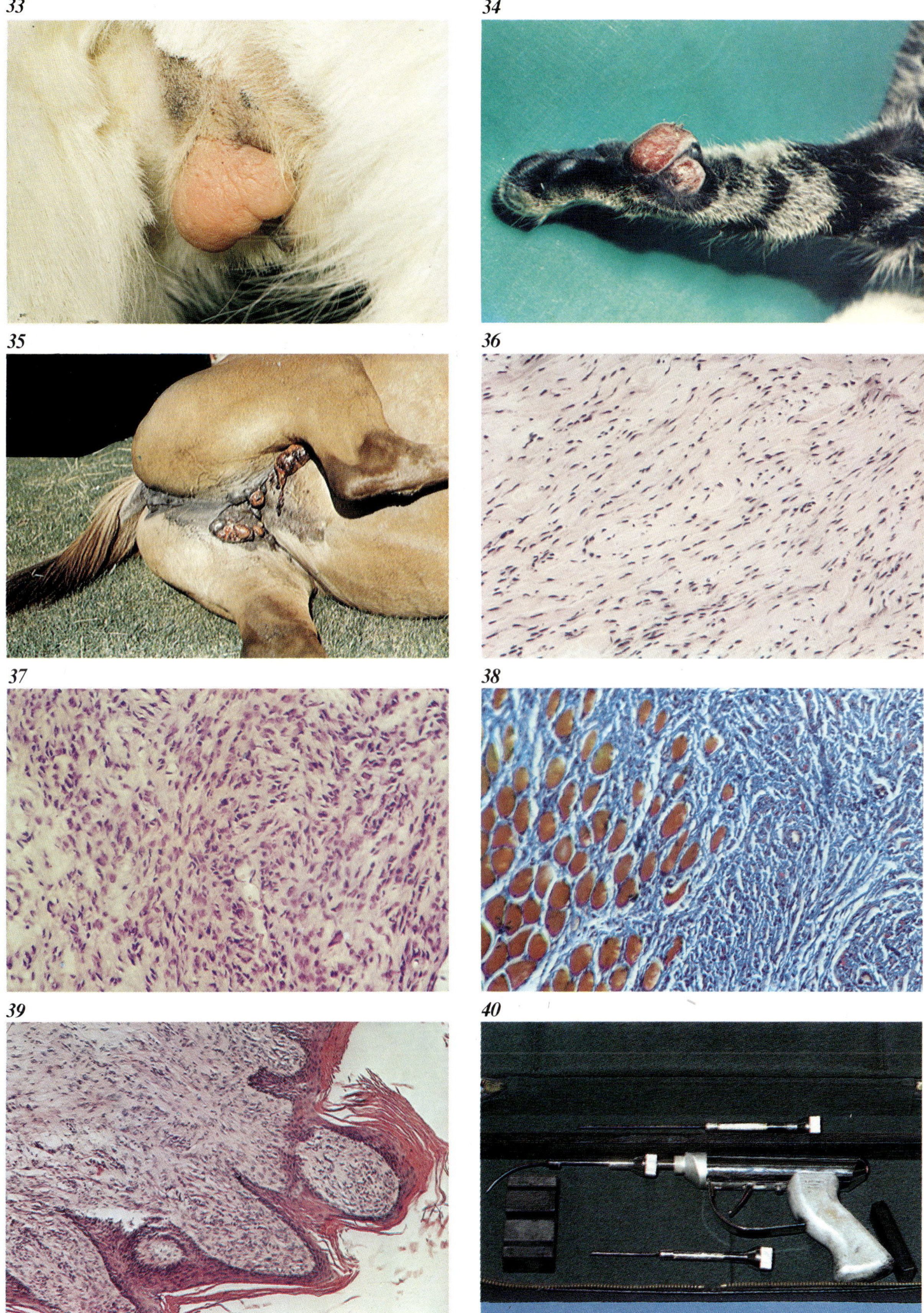
33
34
35
36
37
38
39
40

Aetiology

The aetiology in the dog is unknown, but it has been shown that fibrosarcomas in cats can be caused by an oncorna virus. There have been a number of attempts to transmit equine sarcoids by the use of cell-free extracts but there is as yet no convincing evidence that they are of viral aetiology.

Treatment and prognosis

Fibromas are relatively easy to remove surgically, when the prognosis should be favourable, although local recurrence is seen occasionally, especially after removal of large tumours.

Except for the most poorly differentiated tumours, metastasis from fibrosarcomas of the skin in any species is unusual. Nevertheless the prognosis must be guarded because of the marked tendency towards local recurrence. This is seen most often in the cat but is also a problem in the other species. X-irradiation of the tumour can sometimes be of benefit in the dog and horse, although it seems to be of less value in cats. A dose of 4,000R fractionated X-irradiation can give a complete cure in the dog, especially if treatment is begun soon after surgery and before recurrence is apparent. In the horse, the size, or site of the lesion may preclude complete surgical excision and in these cases irradiation, using radioactive gold seeds can result in a dramatic reduction in tumour volume. The seeds can either be inserted into the mass using a gun (***40***), or applied on a pad to the bed of the lesion following excision of the bulk of the tumour. Total doses up to 5,000R can be used. Treatment is expensive but is often well worthwhile in valuable horses.

Canine Haemangiopericytomas

Occurrence and gross appearance

This tumour is nearly always seen in the subcutaneous tissues of the limbs in middle-aged or older dogs, where it appears grossly as a multilobulated, rather rubbery mass, closely adherent to the skin. There may also be some tendency to invade the deeper tissues. Haemangiopericytomas grow slowly but can become very large if neglected (***41***). The cut surface is firm, pale greyish or yellowish in colour, and fibrous in appearance.

Histological appearance

These tumours are fairly well circumscribed, but not encapsulated, and may sometimes be difficult to distinguish from fibromas or fibrosarcomas. They are composed of small, fusiform cells which are arranged in bundles, or as tight whorls, the characteristic finding being the presence of a small capillary at the centre of the whorl (***42***). The cells usually produce an abundant intercellular collagenous matrix.

Treatment and prognosis

Metastasis is rare and following complete excision the prognosis is good. Very large, diffuse tumours are a problem as they tend to be radio resistant (***43***), so that amputation of the limb may be the only treatment which will result in a complete cure.

Perineural Fibroblastomas (Neurilemmomas, Schwannomas)

Occurrence and gross appearance

Perineural fibroblastomas of the subcutaneous tissues are usually seen in the dog but may occasionally be observed in the other species. In this site the tumours are not obviously associated with nerve trunks and may arise from sensory nerve endings. In gross appearance they resemble canine haemangiopericytomas, usually being found on the limbs, and having a firm, nodular appearance. They are not highly invasive but are closely attached to the surrounding tissues, and have a firm, greyish, fibrous cut surface.

Perineural fibroblastomas arising from large nerve trunks, mainly the brachial plexus, also occur although they are rare. They manifest themselves by neurogenic muscle atrophy or progressive paralysis of the limb and appear grossly as a very firm, well encapsulated, oval thickening of the nerves (***44***). The cut surface is greyish-yellow in colour, homogeneous and fibrous in consistency.

Histological appearance

These tumours show some evidence of local infiltration. They consist of small, spindle-shaped cells, similar to fibrocytes and haemangiopericytes, arranged in wavy bundles or whorls, and producing an intercellular collagenous matrix. Their distinguishing features, however, are the 'palisade' arrangement of the nuclei in some areas and the formation of structures resembling Pacinian corpuscles, consisting of a central, hyaline area surrounded by numerous whorls of tumour cells (***45***).

It should be noted that fibromas, haemangiopericytomas, and subcutaneous perineural fibroblastomas show a close resemblance to each other in gross and histological appearance and also in behaviour. It is thus not always possible to distinguish between them with complete certainty.

Treatment and prognosis

These tumours do not metastasise. The same considerations apply as for haemangiopericytomas.

41 *Large haemangiopericytoma in forelimb of dog.*

42 *Haemangiopericytoma. The characteristic feature is the presence of a capillary at the centre of the concentric whorl of cells. Heidenhain's haematoxylin.*

43 *Extensive ulceration following X-irradiation of haemangiopericytoma to a total of 3,500R.*

44 *Perineural fibroblastoma arising from the brachial plexus in a six-year-old Black Labrador bitch.*

45 *Perineural fibroblastoma of the skin – dog. These tumours contain large relatively acellular whorls resembling Pacinian corpuscles. H & E.*

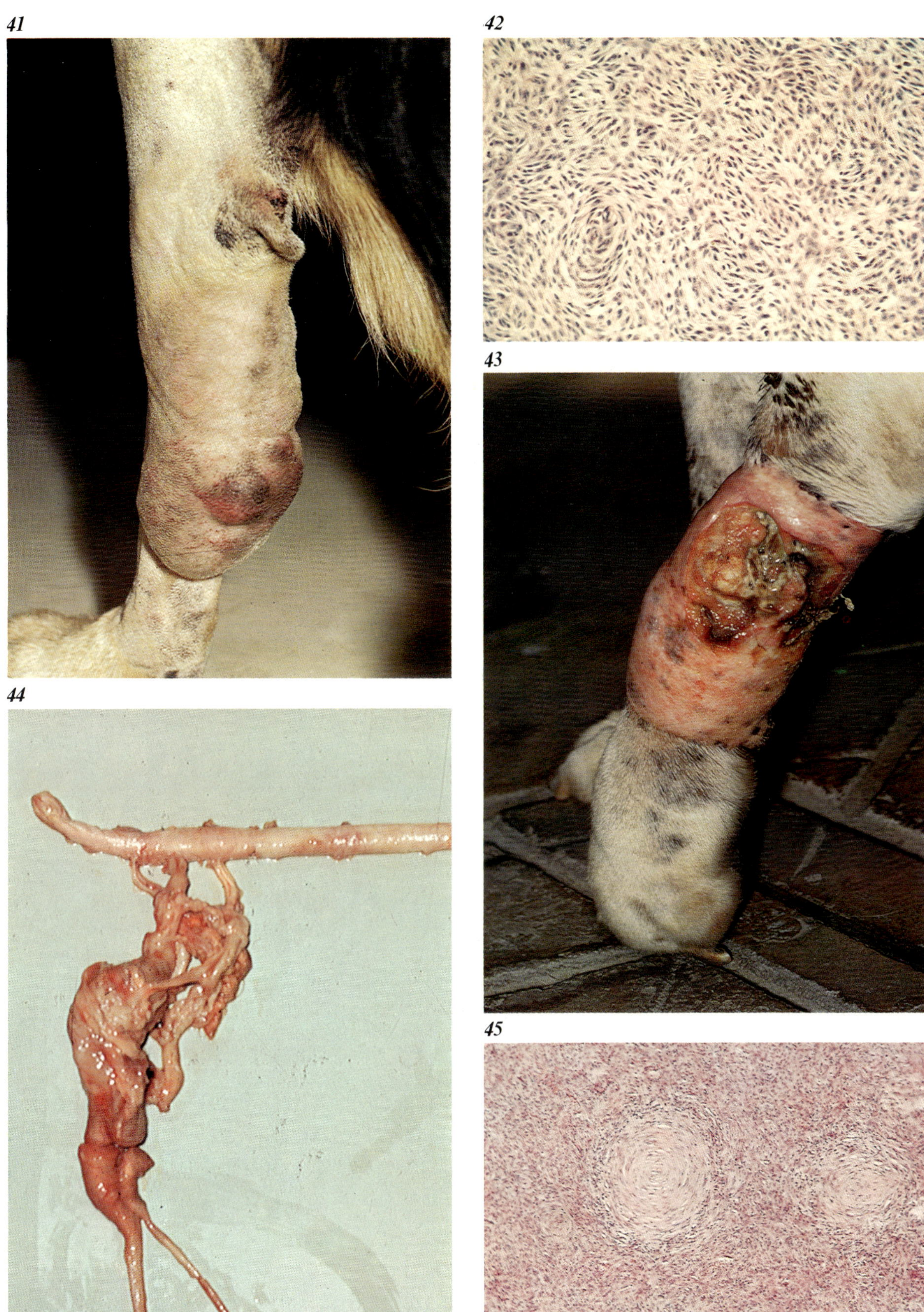
41
42
43
44
45

Cavernous Haemangiomas and Malignant Haemangioendotheliomas (Angiosarcomas)

Occurrence and gross appearance

These neoplasms arise from the endothelium of blood vessels. Benign tumours are seen more commonly than malignant ones, especially in dogs, where they usually occur in the subcutaneous tissues of the back or flanks. They are generally fairly small, measuring from 0.5–2cm in diameter, oval in shape, and well circumscribed. The overlying skin may show loss of hair. In light skinned animals the tumour has a dark reddish appearance and, if it ulcerates, may bleed profusely. The cut surface of the fresh tumour is dark red in colour, intensely congested and, if washed well, has an appearance resembling a tiny honeycomb.

Malignant haemangioendotheliomas are rapidly growing and highly invasive tumours which become very large and quickly ulcerate through the skin. They are friable, with a surface mottled by irregular areas of haemorrhage and necrosis (***46***). The differential diagnosis is from exuberant granulation tissue.

Histological appearance

Cavernous haemangiomas are well circumscribed but not encapsulated, and are situated in the dermal connective tissues. They consist of regular, cystic spaces, separated from each other by mature collagen fibres, lined by a single layer of endothelial cells and filled with normal red cells (***47***).

Malignant haemangioendotheliomas are poorly circumscribed, very invasive, and consist of hyperchromatic oval cells, lining irregular sinusoidal spaces containing red cells (***48***). Mitotic figures are seen commonly and in the less well differentiated tumours the cells are packed closely together with little evidence of blood filled spaces.

Treatment and prognosis

Surgical removal of cavernous haemangiomas leads to a complete cure. Haemangioendotheliomas are extremely difficult to remove surgically, usually recur locally, and readily metastasise (***49***). Thus the prognosis for animals with these tumours should always be very guarded.

Lipomas and Liposarcomas

Occurrence and gross appearance

These tumours are seen most often in dogs, less frequently in cats, and rarely in horses. Benign tumours are much more common than malignant ones, and are seen especially in obese, middle-aged or older bitches, where they develop in the subcutaneous fat of the flanks, chest, pre-sternal area, axilla, and groin (***50***).

They appear clinically as soft, well circumscribed and very mobile tumours, sometimes feeling almost cystic on palpation. They may become very large but the overlying skin is unaffected and does not ulcerate. Most appear grossly as well circumscribed spheres of apparently normal fat (***51***), with a whitish homogeneous cut surface (***52***), but some infiltrate widely between muscles.

Liposarcomas are rare tumours in the skin. They develop in similar sites to lipomas, but are very invasive, so that they appear as firm, adherent masses, quickly leading to ulceration of the epidermis. Their gross appearance may not at first suggest their tissue of origin, since they tend to have a firm, greyish, well vascularised cut surface, and their true nature is frequently only revealed histologically.

Histological appearance

Lipomas are well circumscribed and surrounded by a thin fibrous capsule. They consist of a closely packed sheet of very large cells with clearly defined cytoplasmic boundaries, but in paraffin sections the cytoplasm appears to consist of an empty space. Nuclei are small, intensely basophilic, and pushed to the periphery of the cell (***53***). Liposarcomas are diffusely invasive, and consist of polygonal or spherical cells with large open nuclei, amongst which mitotic figures are seen frequently. They are well vascularized, and the cells contain a variable number of intracytoplasmic fat vacuoles (***54***).

Aetiology

The observation that lipomas are seen mainly in obese animals, suggests that they may follow hyperplasia of fat cells.

Treatment and prognosis

Surgical removal of even large subcutaneous lipomas is frequently simple. In some dogs several months of strict dieting prior to surgical intervention has reduced the volume of the tumour which has then been easily excised. Lipomas which develop within deeper tissues and infiltrate between muscle bundles may recur locally because of the difficulty of ensuring complete excision.

The prognosis for animals with liposarcomas should always be guarded since these tumours usually recur locally and metastasise to the lungs.

46 *Malignant haemangioendothelioma in the forelimb of a nine-year-old Labrador Retriever.*

47 *Cavernous haemangioma – dog. H & E.*

48 *Malignant haemangioendothelioma – dog. H & E.*

49 *Multiple pulmonary secondaries from malignant haemangioendothelioma of the skin – dog.*

50 *Large subcutaneous lipoma in the groin of an old Labrador Retriever. This tumour had been enlarging slowly for several years.*

51 *Subcutaneous lipoma – dog. Note the obvious capsule which renders surgical excision relatively easy.*

52 *Cut surface of lipomas showing their resemblance to normal fat – dog.*

53 *Lipoma – dog. The nuclei are very small, hyperchromatic and pushed to the edge of the cell. H & E.*

54 *Liposarcoma. The cells are very active and have abundant cytoplasm containing variably sized fat droplets. H & E.*

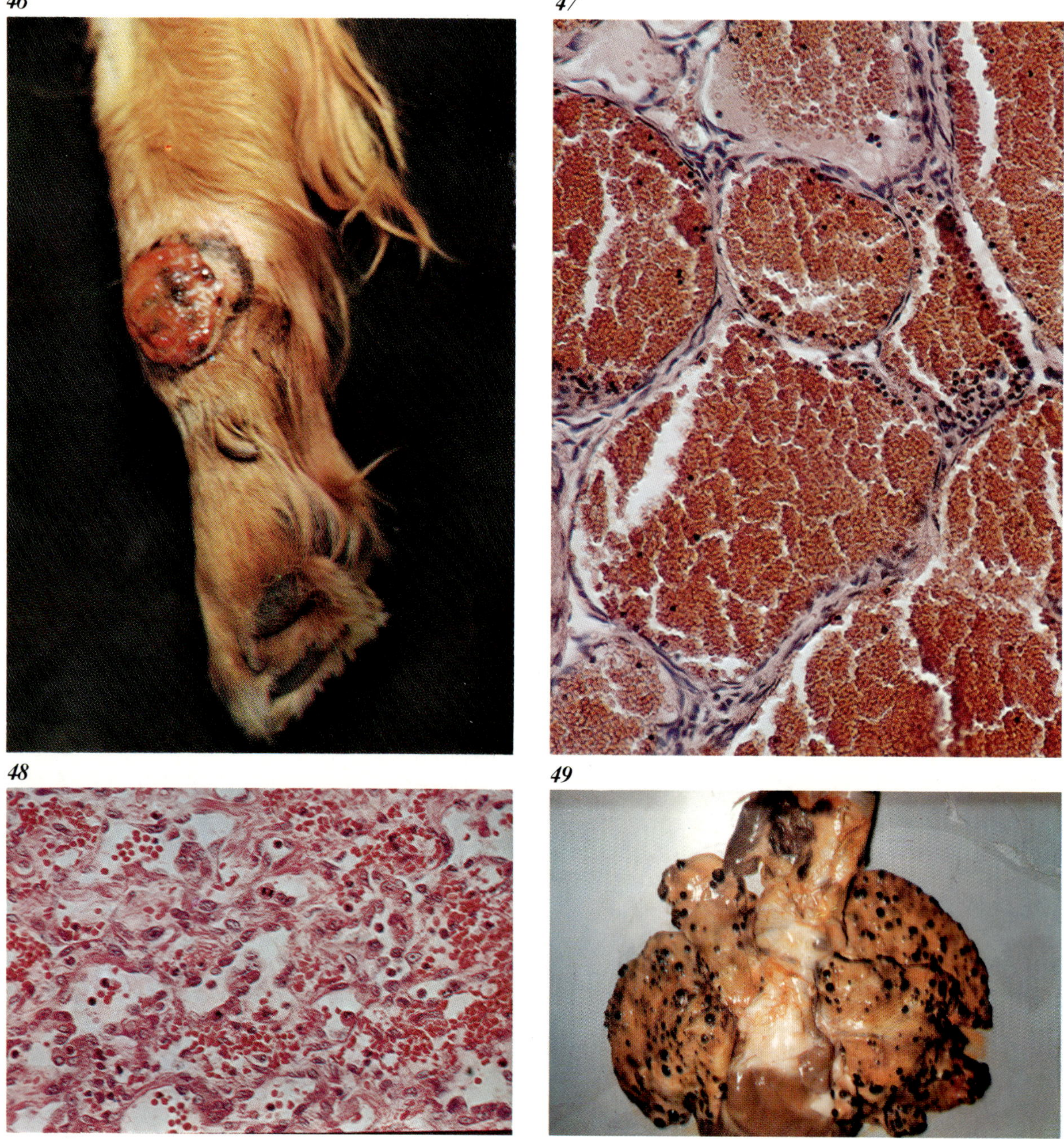

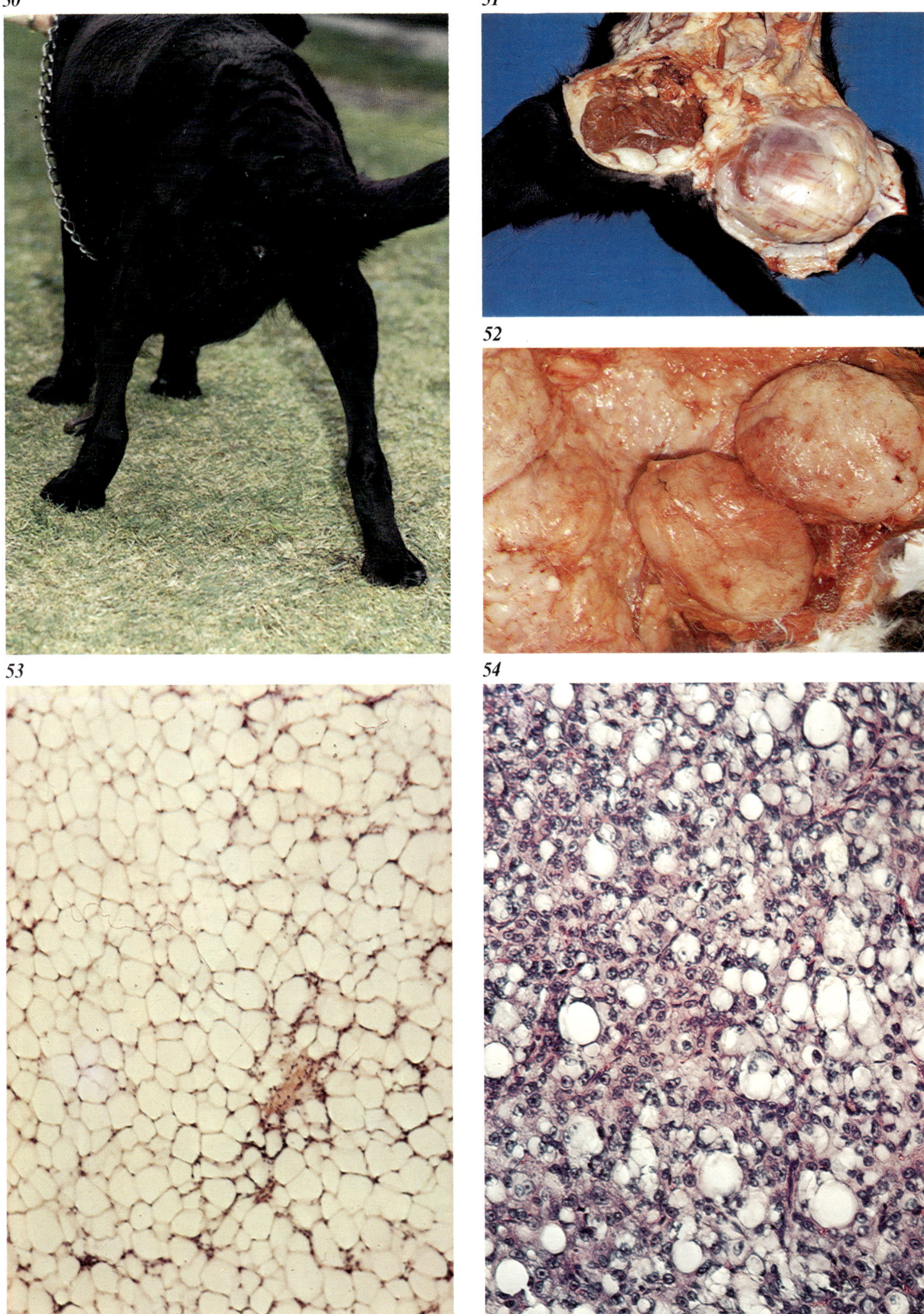
50
51
52
53
54

Mastocytomas

Occurrence and gross appearance

Mastocytomas are of most significance in the dog, where they account for about 10% of the total number of skin tumours. They are found infrequently in cats, and rarely in horses. In dogs there is a marked breed incidence, with Boxers and Boston Terriers being most frequently affected. Labradors and Retrievers also develop them commonly but they are seen rarely in Poodles and Hounds. Mastocytomas can occur anywhere in the skin, and there appears to be little predilection for any particular site. In dogs they can be either single or multiple and vary from slowly growing, soft and flabby tumours, to rapidly growing, firm, multinodular masses which invade the skin and cause ulceration and local irritation (***55***). Their cut surface is usually yellowish brown or greenish in colour and may be mottled by haemorrhage. They are never encapsulated but the slowly growing tumours are more defined than the rapidly growing ones. In the cat mastocytomas tend to be small (*usually less than 0.5cm in diameter*) but multiple throughout the skin (***56***).

Histological appearance

These tumours are non-encapsulated and consist of a diffuse infiltration of the dermal connective tissues by masses of mast cells, amongst which eosinophil polymorphs are scattered in varying numbers. There is a considerable variation in the degree of differentiation of the mast cells in dogs and tumours have been divided into three grades, which have been shown to be of prognostic significance. The best differentiated tumours consist of relatively small numbers of mast cells with abundant, purplish cytoplasm and a central spherical nucleus (***57***). Mitotic figures are rare, and the cells may appear to be separated by large empty spaces. Poorly differentiated tumours consist of closely packed cells, with a large, irregular nucleus, sparse cytoplasm, and numerous mitoses (***58***).

Mastocytomas in the cat have a somewhat different appearance. They consist of fairly well differentiated mast cells, arranged as a homogeneous, closely packed sheet, amongst which eosinophil polymorphs are not conspicuous. These tumours can be diagnosed rapidly by staining impression smears, fixed in ethanol, in 1% toluidine blue. Mast cells contain metachromatically staining substances which appear as multiple, bright red or purple granules in the cytoplasm (***59***).

Aetiology

Mast cell leukaemias in the dog have been transmitted using cell-free extracts. Transmission studies using extracts from solid mastocytomas in the dog and cat, however, failed to produce tumours.

Treatment and prognosis

In dogs slowly growing, well differentiated mastocytomas are easily removed surgically, following which more than 80% of animals are completely cured. Less well differentiated tumours have a marked tendency towards local recurrence and metastasis to regional lymph nodes and carry a guarded prognosis. Following surgical excision, over 70% of animals with poorly differentiated tumours have to be destroyed because of regrowth; the mean survival time post operatively being only 18 weeks. Mastocytomas are radiosensitive and following excision of the more malignant tumours fractionated X-irradiation, before tumour recurrence, is advisable. A significant prolongation of life can be achieved even in animals with regional lymph node metastasis following fractionated X-irradiation to a total tumour dose of 3,000–3,500R. Useful, although temporary regressions can also be obtained using a combination of cyclophosphamide (*1–2mg/kg*) and prednisolone (*2mg/kg*) orally every other day.

The prognosis in cats with mastocytomas should always be guarded because of the frequency with which the tumour becomes generalised.

Reticulum Cell Sarcomas

Occurrence and gross appearance

Reticulum cell sarcomas are seen almost exclusively in middle-aged or older dogs, and may be found anywhere in the skin, with a propensity for the flanks, head and limbs. They vary in size from a few millimetres to several centimetres in diameter and are rapidly growing tumours which quickly ulcerate through the overlying epidermis (***60***) and infiltrate into the surrounding tissues.

Histological appearance

These tumours are often difficult to distinguish from histiocytomas, although they tend to be larger. They consist of a closely packed, non-circumscribed sheet of large cells, with an irregularly shaped, indented nucleus, and indistinct cell boundaries (***61***). Mitotic figures are common and staining for reticulin reveals an abundant network of fine fibrils investing individual or small groups of cells (***62***).

Treatment and prognosis

The tumours are closely attached to the skin, but not to the underlying tissues, and are easily removed when they are small. Although they appear histologically to be highly malignant, like histiocytomas, they do not often behave in this way. Local recurrence and regional lymph node metastasis can present a problem following surgical removal of larger tumours, but fractionated X-irradiation to a total dose of 3,000R will produce dramatic regression in most of these cases, with the possibility of a complete cure.

Histiocytomas

Occurrence and gross appearance

These common tumours are confined to the dog. They are nearly always solitary and are found between four months and three years of age, although older animals can be affected. They usually occur on the ear flaps or distal extremities but can be seen elsewhere, and have a history of very rapid growth, reaching their maximum size of 1–2cm diameter in about three weeks. The overlying hair is lost and the epidermis becomes ulcerated so that they appear as well circumscribed dome shaped lesions, which are freely movable over the underlying tissues (***63***).

Histological appearance

The tumour consists of a diffuse infiltration of the dermal connective tissues and overlying epidermis by masses of histiocytic cells, having a large, often indented nucleus and abundant cytoplasm (***64***). Cytoplasmic boundaries are indistinct, and mitotic figures are seen commonly. A variable number of lymphocytes are seen scattered amongst the histiocytes and in some tumours, appear to predominate.

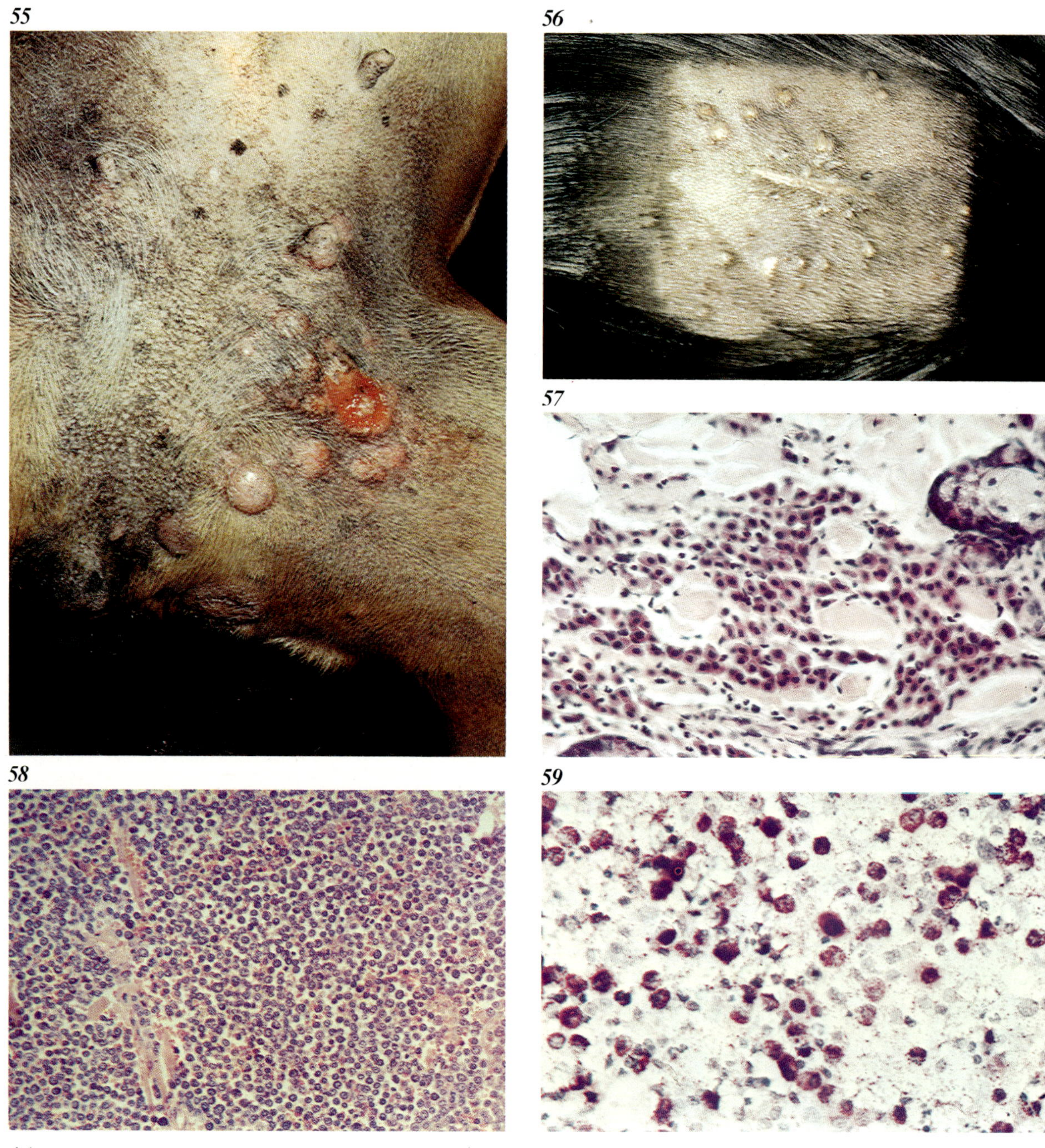

55 *56* *57* *58* *59*

55 Multinodular, invasive mastocytoma in an eight-year-old Boxer. This appearance is indicative of malignancy and carries a poor prognosis.

56 Multiple discrete mastocytomas in a cat. A biopsy scar is visible in the centre of the shaved area.

57 Well differentiated mastocytoma – dog. H & E.

58 Poorly differentiated mastocytoma – dog. The cytoplasm is sparse and mitotic figures may be common. H & E.

59 Impression smear of mastocytoma stained with toluidine blue. Note the purple staining metachromatic granules in the cytoplasm of the mast cells – dog.

60 Reticulum cell sarcoma on the forefoot of a five-year-old Terrier.

61 Reticulum cell sarcoma. H & E.

62 Reticulum cell sarcoma stained for reticulin. Fine black fibrils are seen investing small clumps of cells or individual cells themselves. Gomori's silver impregnation.

63 Histiocytoma – eight-months-old Collie.

64 Histiocytoma. These tumours are very active and have a definitely malignant histological appearance. H & E.

60

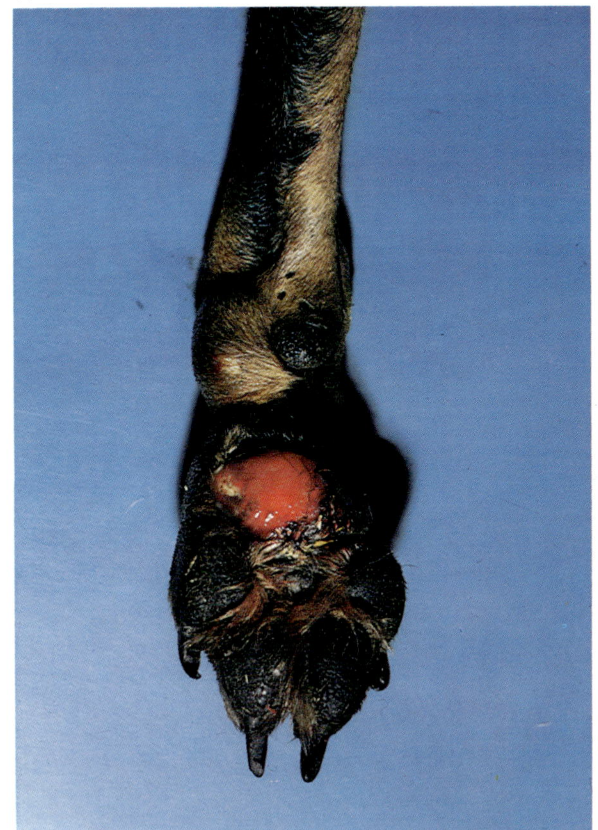

61

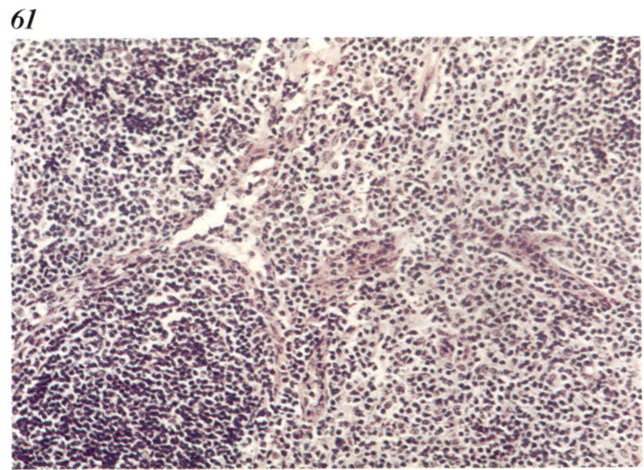

62

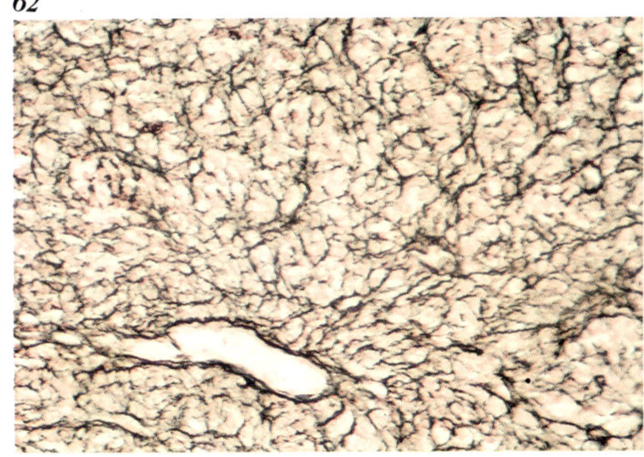

63

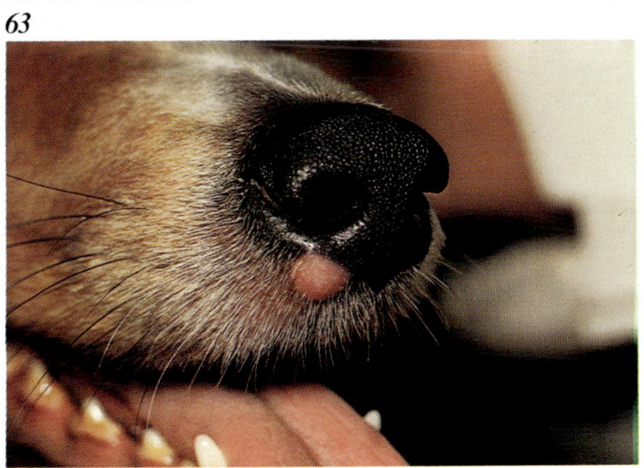

64

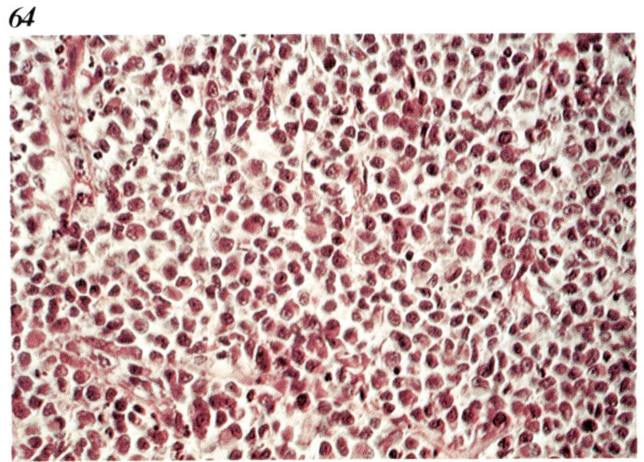

Aetiology

The natural history of these tumours suggests that they are of viral aetiology, but transmission experiments, using cell-free extracts, have so far failed to prove this.

Treatment and prognosis

If these tumours are untreated they regress spontaneously within three to six months. Surgical removal is usually completely successful but, rarely, local recurrence is seen. The tumours are very radiosensitive and the prognosis is always good.

NON-NEOPLASTIC TUMOUR-LIKE LESIONS OF THE SKIN

Calcinosis Circumscripta

Occurrence and gross appearance

This condition, which is frequently confused with neoplastic disease, is seen only in dogs, especially those under two years of age. Large dogs, particularly Alsatians and Wolfhounds are most frequently affected but it can occur in smaller breeds. The lesion consists of a firm, well circumscribed, painless mass or masses in the deeper tissues of the subcutis over one of the limb joints, or in the tissues of the tongue. The radiographic appearance is quite typical, the mass appearing as a well-defined, intensely radiopaque structure which is clearly not attached to the bone (***65***). The cut surface is also characteristic, being very gritty, and consisting of numerous small, irregular foci of chalky, whitish material separated by firm fibrous septa (***66***). When these lesions are cut and fixed, the fixative becomes 'milky' in appearance.

Histological appearance

Each nodule is composed of a dense stroma of mature, acellular collagen which contains numerous foci of structureless calcified débris. Between this material and the fibrous tissue, a very narrow zone of calcifying macrophages and foreign body giant cells may be discernible (***67***).

Aetiology

Although the mechanism whereby the lesions develop is unknown, the marked breed predisposition of the condition suggests that it has a genetic basis.

Treatment and prognosis

If these masses are left in situ the overlying skin may ulcerate to produce a chronic discharging sinus. Surgical excision is usually simple although local recurrence, especially in the tongue, can be troublesome. The lesions generally cease to develop when the animal reaches maturity.

Cysts

Occurrence and gross appearance

The most commonly occurring cysts are those which develop from the epidermis in dogs, and, less frequently, cats. The usual site is in the skin of the back, shoulders and flanks, or between the toes. Cysts on the body generally measure from 1–2cm in diameter, but can occasionally be much larger, and may be multiple. They develop slowly, eventually manifesting themselves as rubbery, well circumscribed masses in the superficial tissues of the dermis. If left untreated they lose their overlying hair and finally rupture, discharging a whitish, greasy, structureless material. Their cut surface consists of a central mass of greasy débris, sometimes containing hairs, surrounded by a fibrous capsule (***68***).

Sebaceous cysts are much less common but have a similar gross appearance. Interdigital cysts occur commonly in dogs, are frequently multiple, develop rapidly, and

65 *Radiograph of calcinosis circumscripta over the elbow joint in a young Alsatian (German Shepherd). The mass is not attached to the underlying bone.*

66 *Calcinosis circumscripta – cut surface. Note the chalky white foci of calcified necrotic debris.*

67 *Calcinosis circumscripta. The zone of necrosis is surrounded by a thin rim of giant cells and macrophages. H & E.*

68 *Epidermal cyst – cut surface.*

69 *Multiple interdigital cysts.*

70 *Epidermal cyst. The cyst lining is a well differentiated stratified squamous epithelium. H & E.*

71 *Dermoid cyst containing hair shafts which are growing into the central lumen.*

72 *Epidermal cyst with neoplastic transformation of the epithelium to produce a well differentiated squamous cell carcinoma.*

73 *Inter-digital cyst showing infiltration of the surrounding connective tissues by chronic inflammatory cells. H & E.*

74 *Sebaceous cyst. H & E.*

75 *Wall of pigmented cyst from the skin of the ventral neck in a dog. Many cells contain melanin granules in their cytoplasm.*

65

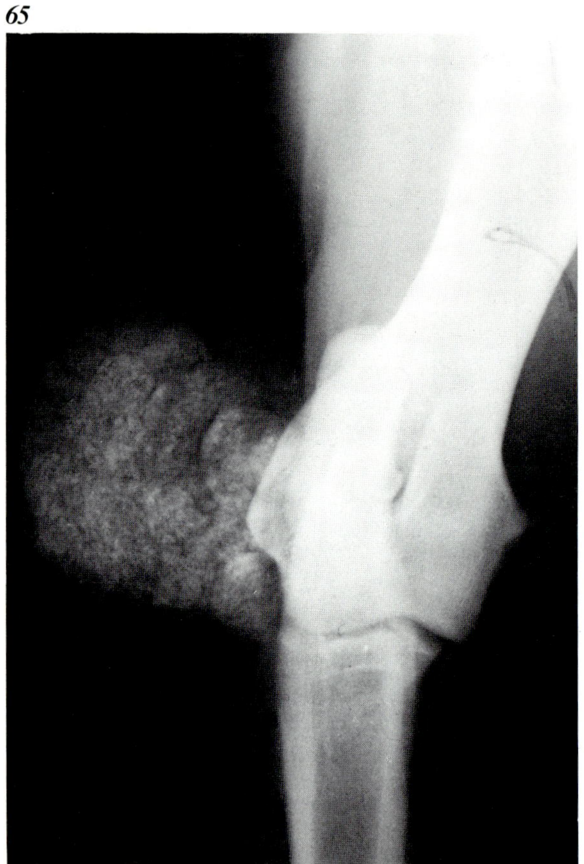

66

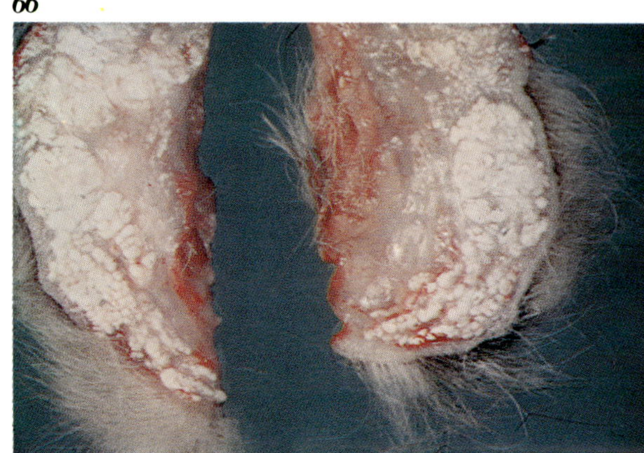

67

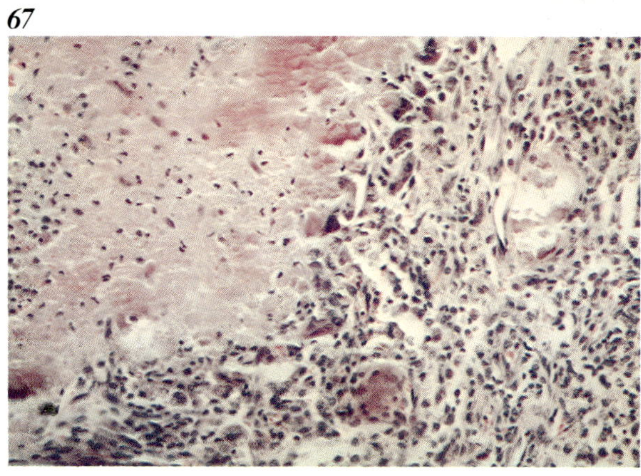

68

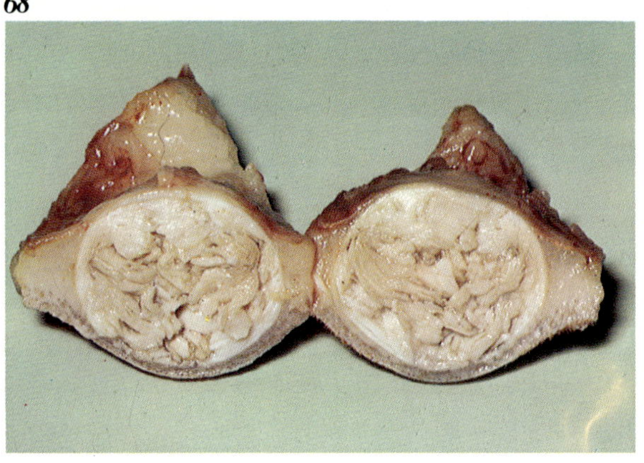

69

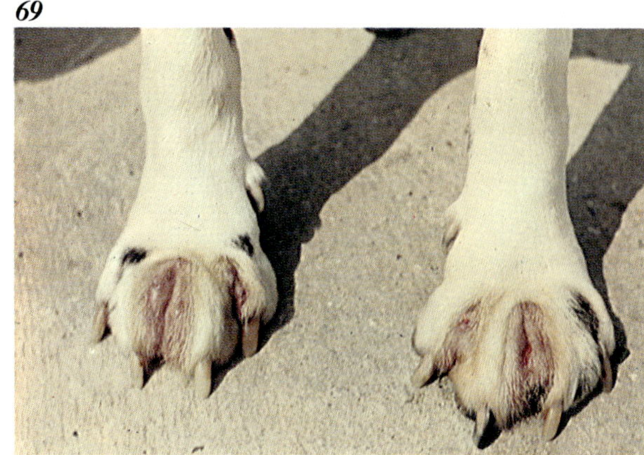

cause considerable irritation. This leads to licking and biting, so that ulceration of the overlying skin, with secondary infection, is usual (***69***).

Intensely pigmented cysts, which may measure several centimetres in diameter and which are filled with a coal black fluid are occasionally seen in the skin in both dogs and cats. Small masses composed of a number of thin walled cysts, filled with a clear fluid, and probably derived from sweat glands are also found in dogs.

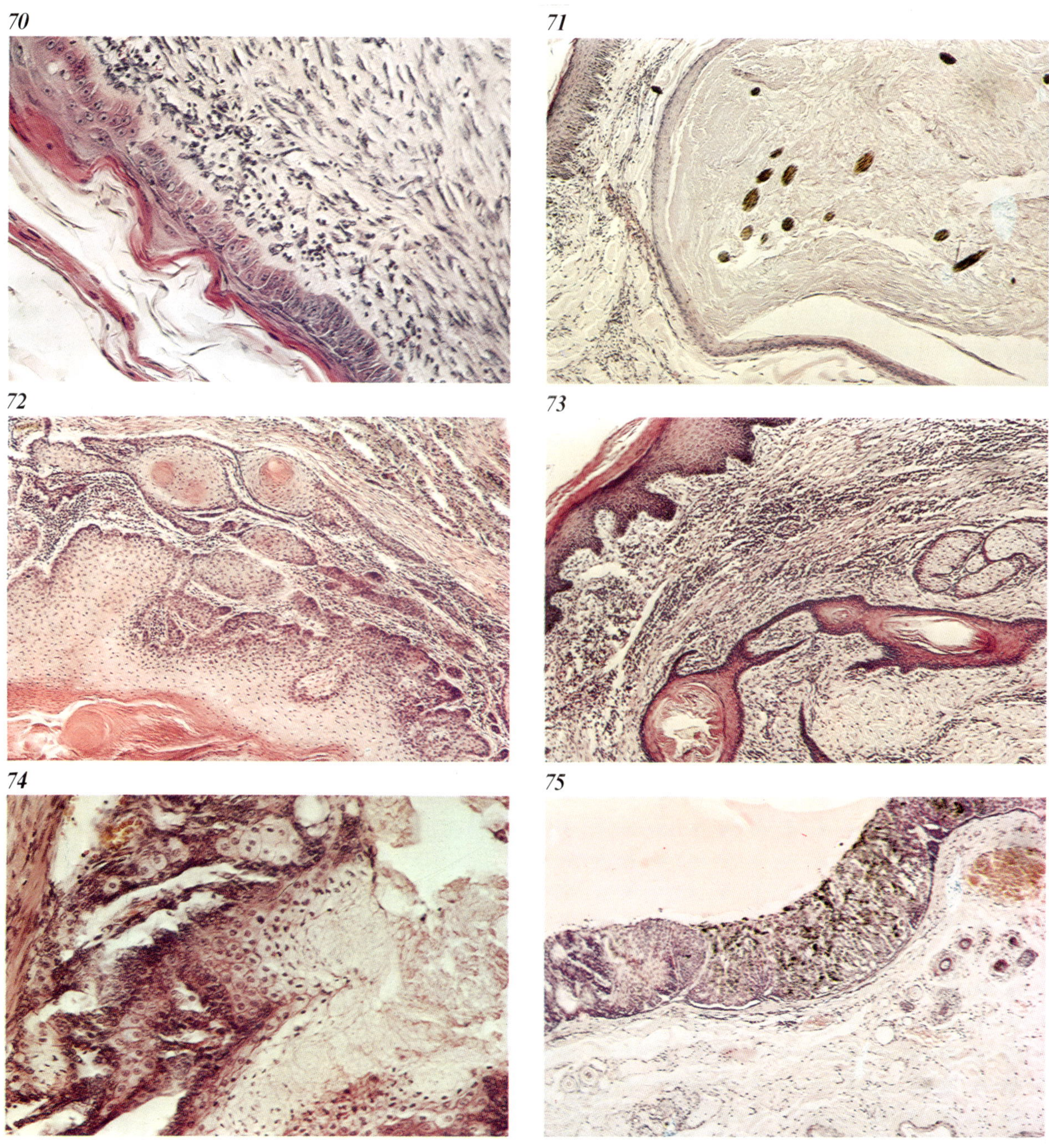

Histological appearance

All cysts are well circumscribed and encapsulated. Epidermal cysts are composed of a dense central mass of keratin, which is often arranged in concentric whorls, and surrounded by a thin, well differentiated stratified squamous epithelium (*70*). In some cases this epithelium contains hair follicles, which are sending hairs into the central lumen (*71*), the structure then being a dermoid cyst.

Many epidermal cysts are complex, being composed of a number of closely packed cystic structures, and in some there is evidence of true neoplastic transformation of the epithelium (*72*).

Interdigital cysts have a very similar appearance to epidermal cysts, but are usually surrounded by masses of inflammatory cells, indicating rupture into the surrounding tissues (*73*). Sebaceous cysts are lined by several layers of cells undergoing sebaceous differentiation (*74*).

The unusual, intensely pigmented cysts seen in dogs and cats are composed of a lining membrane of large, hyperchromatic, columnar cells arranged in chains or thrown up into branching, ingrowing papillae. The cells themselves are packed with melanin granules (*75*), and the large central lumen is filled with this pigment in some cases.

Aetiology

Cysts without true hairs are said to develop as a result of blockage of sebaceous ducts or hair follicles, whilst those which are producing hairs are believed to be due to inclusion of a portion of the skin below the epidermis, perhaps following trauma. Dogs which develop interdigital cysts may have a genetic tendency to do so, whilst the origin and cause of pigmented cysts remain obscure, although they may be an unusual form of basal cell tumour.

Treatment and prognosis

The prognosis is good following surgical removal even in cysts showing evidence of neoplastic transformation. Incision and cautery of interdigital cysts is successful but further cysts may occur between other toes.

Granulomas

Occurrence and gross appearance

Up to 14% of lesions removed from the skin and suspected of being neoplastic are found histologically to be granulomas or other chronic inflammatory lesions. In general granulomas tend to develop relatively slowly and appear as ulcerated lesions which are closely attached to the skin, and may also involve the underlying tissues (*76*). They are usually impossible to distinguish from true neoplasms on gross examination (*77*).

Histological appearance

The appearance of these lesions varies somewhat with the causative agent, but basically they consist of masses of macrophages, in some cases forming syncytia and giant cells (*78*), surrounded by a zone of lymphocytes and proliferating fibroblasts. Zones of necrosis are often found, especially in granulomas of bacterial aetiology, for example those caused by atypical acid and alcohol fast organisms in the cat (*79 and 80*). Some chronic inflammatory lesions contain areas composed almost entirely of rapidly proliferating, thin walled blood vessels (***81***) and great care must be taken to distinguish these from malignant haemangioendotheliomas.

Aetiology

In addition to bacteria and fungi there are a variety of aetiological agents which lead to the formation of granulomas, perhaps the commonest being foreign bodies which penetrate the skin. Granulomas may also be caused by parasites, for example warble fly larvae in horses and demodectic mange mites in dogs. Chronic trauma, as in 'lick granulomas' in dogs (***76***) and cats, is a major cause of skin lesions in animals.

Treatment and prognosis

In most granulomas the best form of treatment is surgical excision, following which a complete recovery is to be expected. 'Lick granulomas' in dogs can be treated with corticosteroids and bandaging, but surgical excision is of little value unless self inflicted trauma can be prevented during healing. Radiotherapy to a total dose of 2,500R has been used with some success, apparently because pruritus is relieved and healing can take place.

77 *Granuloma on penis of dog.*

78 *Foreign body granuloma – skin of dog. This was induced by subcutaneous injection of an oily compound, droplets of which can be seen within some giant cells. H & E.*

79 *Subcutaneous granuloma in cat due to atypical acid fast bacteria. H & E.*

80 *Acid and alcohol fast bacteria within macrophages. Mycobacterial granuloma on a cat's skin. Ziehl Neelsen stain.*

81 *Chronic inflammatory lesion in a dog resembling haemangioendothelioma. There is usually a marked fibrous reaction in addition to the capillary proliferation. H & E.*

76 *'Lick' granuloma in skin of forelimb – five-year-old dog.*

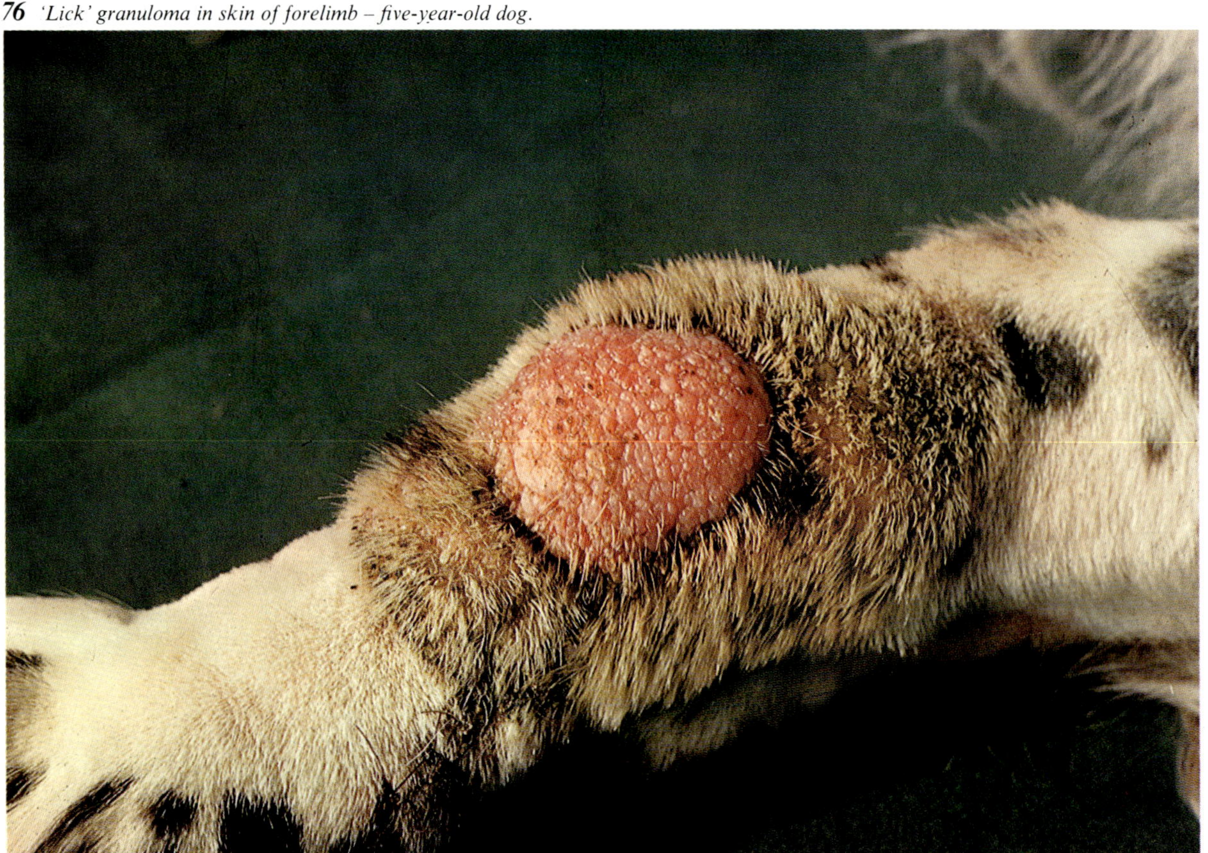

77

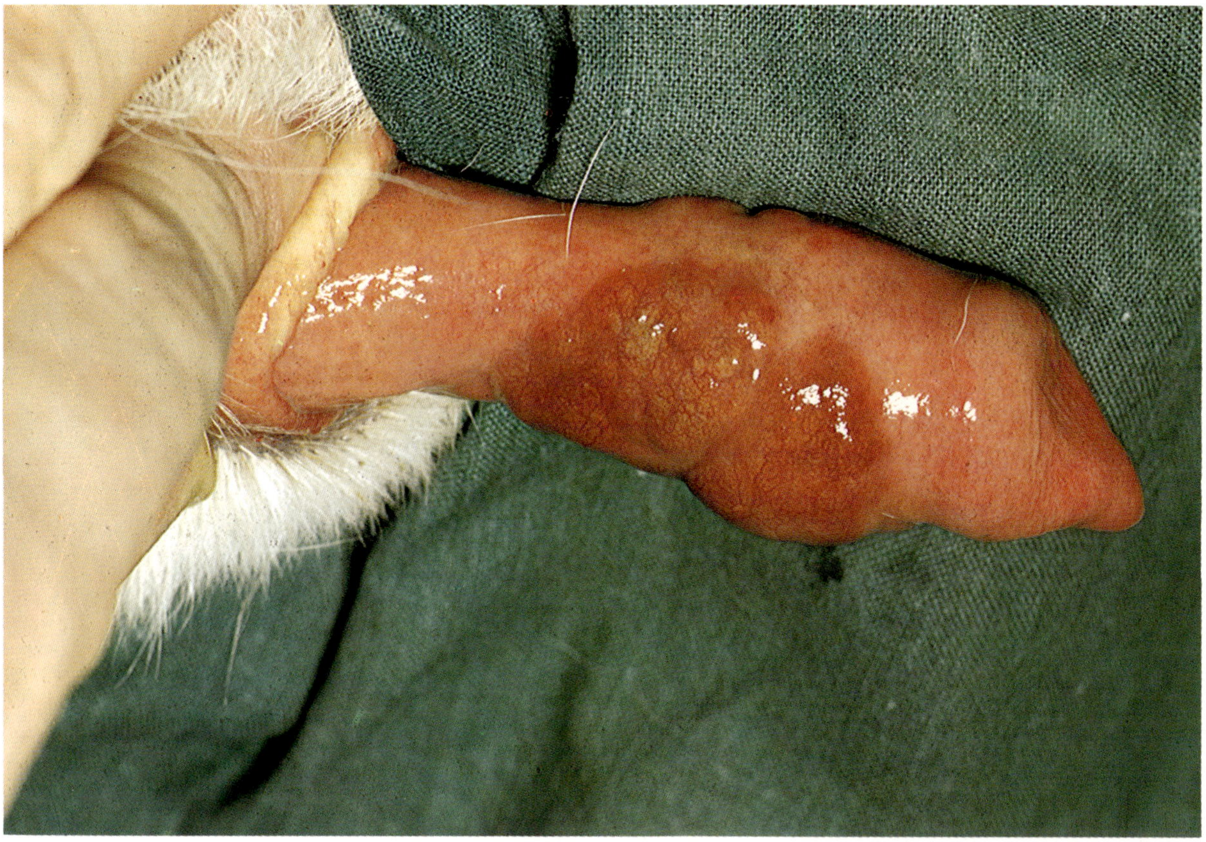

78

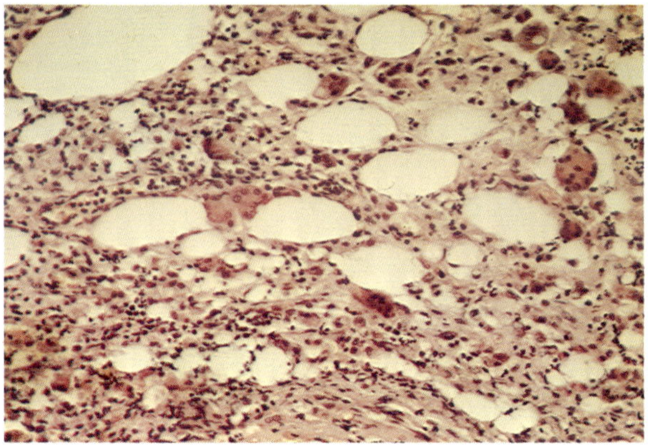

79

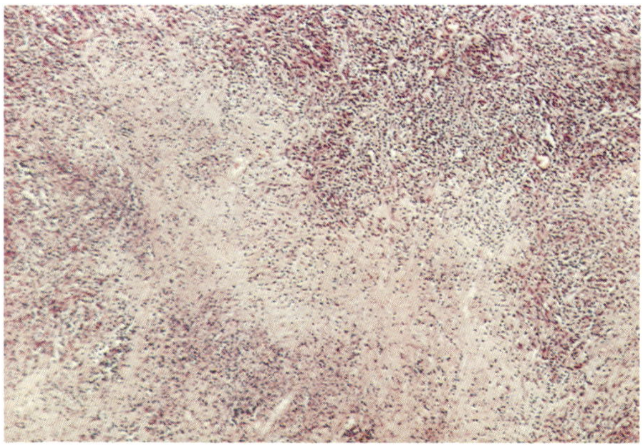

80

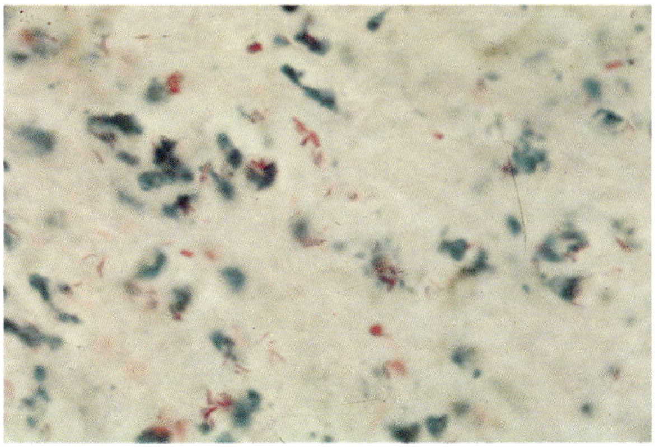

81

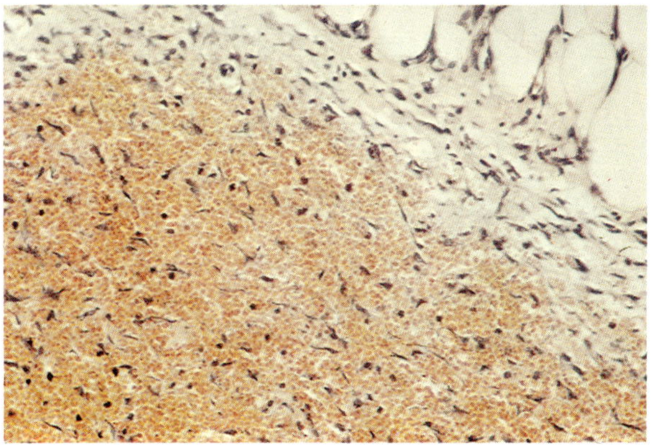

Chapter 2
The Mammary Glands

Mammary tumours are extremely rare in the horse, but are the commonest single group of neoplasms in the bitch, accounting for approximately 25% of all tumours. They are also relatively common in cats, but are seen less frequently than skin tumours in this species.

In dogs, the commonest neoplasm is the mixed mammary tumour, which is usually benign. Carcinomas are also relatively common, whilst adenomas, sarcomas and mixed carcino-sarcomas are observed less often. Histologically, malignant tumours in dogs represent about 50% of the total number, but metastasis does not occur in all these cases. Malignant tumours appear more frequently in the two posterior mammary glands (*by convention designated glands 4 and 5*) than in the anterior glands.

When spaying is performed before the 2nd oestrus cycle in the bitch there is a marked decrease in the incidence of mammary neoplasia, but spaying performed after this time does not affect subsequent tumour development.

In cats, more than 95% of mammary tumours are carcinomas and the mixed mammary tumour does not occur. Tumours can be seen in any mammary gland and show no preference for the inguinal region.

Benign Mixed Mammary Tumours

Occurrence and gross appearance

These tumours are found only in the dog, usually in middle-aged or older bitches and often develop in several glands at the same time. When seen they are of variable size, and are characteristically firm and knobbly in consistency, well circumscribed, and freely mobile (***82***). The overlying skin does not ulcerate except in the larger tumours, where it probably does so due to external trauma. Mixed tumours tend to be very slow growing but may increase considerably in size in the immediately post oestrus period, regressing incompletely during anoestrus. Their cut surface is dark in colour, may be bony, and sometimes contains sheets of bluish, translucent cartilage or small, fluid filled cysts.

Very rarely these tumours are seen in old male dogs.

Histological appearance

This is extremely variable, but a number of features tend to be more or less uniform. These tumours are well circumscribed, surrounded by a thin fibrous capsule and composed of both epithelial and mesenchymal elements which are usually well differentiated. The epithelial component consists of regular acinar structures lined by a single layer of cuboidal epithelial cells frequently containing a hyaline, eosinophilic secretion. The commonest mesenchymal component is myxomatous tissue which can be found as small foci of polygonal cells, separated from each other by an abundant mucinous stroma. Tumours containing only myxomatous and epithelial elements are referred to as complex adenomas (***83***). Other common mesenchymal components include sheets of mature cartilage, areas of cancellous bone sometimes containing marrow cavities and areas of proliferating fibroblasts. It is not unusual to have all these components in the same tumour (***84***), but one type usually predominates. In some tumours it seems that there is a mesenchymal component, e.g. cartilage, myxomatous tissue, fibrous tissue, or bone, without any evidence of an epithelial element. This type of tumour may be classified as a chondroma, myxoma (***85***), fibroma or osteoma, but if a search of the entire mass is made, a few acini will usually be found, and all these lesions should probably be classified as mixed mammary tumours.

Aetiology

The observation that these tumours grow most rapidly in the immediate post oestrus period suggests that they are under hormonal control, but the exact nature of this is not known.

Treatment and prognosis

Although these tumours are slowly growing and apparently innocuous, the affected mammary gland should be excised as soon as possible because of the possibility of malignant transformation. Following early excision, the prognosis is good.

Sarcomas

Occurrence and gross appearance

An unknown but possibly high percentage of benign mixed tumours in dogs will undergo malignant transformation if left untreated. When this occurs, the small, slowly growing tumour rapidly enlarges, ulcerates through the overlying skin (***86***) and infiltrates the underlying tissues. Sarcomatous tumours may also develop without passing through a recognisable benign mixed stage, being rapidly growing and invasive from the start.

Histological appearance

There is considerable histological variation in these neoplasms. In most cases only one tissue becomes malignant, although occasionally true carcinosarcomas, in which both mesenchymal and epithelial elements are malignant are seen. In cases where transformation has occurred fairly recently the tumour may contain remnants of an original mixed tumour, but in advanced cases the malignant element usually obliterates this, so that the tumour appears as a fibrosarcoma (***87***), osteosarcoma, chondrosarcoma, liposarcoma or myxosarcoma.

Treatment and prognosis

A radiograph of the thorax to detect metastatic spread to the lungs is made. All round opacities with a diameter greater than 8mm are suspect (***88***) as are diffuse opacities (***89***). If there is no radiographic evidence of secondary spread mastectomy is performed without delay. Because of the lymph drainage system (***90***) it is recommended that when a tumour occurs in one of the anterior three glands mastectomy of all three glands should be carried out and if tumours occur in glands 4 or 5 both of these mammae should be excised. Superficial inguinal, popliteal and axillary lymph nodes are also excised if they are visibly or palpably enlarged. Metastasis to the regional lymph nodes and lungs is common with sarcomas (***91** and **92***), as is local recurrence, so that the prognosis should be guarded.

X-irradiation is of little value in the treatment, or prevention of recurrence, of mammary tumours. Hormones related to testosterone (*e.g. Drostanolone Propionate*) are of doubtful value in producing regression but because of their anabolic action may effect a temporary improvement in the general condition of the animal.

82 *Benign mixed mammary tumour – dog.*

83 *Complex mammary adenoma showing only epithelial and myxomatous elements. H & E.*

84 *Benign mixed mammary tumour showing epithelial and mesenchymal elements. H & E.*

85 *Myxoma in canine mammary gland. Heidenhain's haematoxylin.*

86 *Large fibrosarcoma, developing from a mixed mammary tumour.*

87 *Mammary fibrosarcoma. H & E.*

88 *Radiograph of lung metastases from a mammary osteosarcoma in a 10-year-old bitch.*

89 *Radiograph of diffuse lung opacities in a dog. These were produced by multiple small secondaries from an adenocarcinoma of the mammary gland.*

90 *Mammary lymphatic drainage in the dog.*

91 *Lung metastases from a malignant mammary tumour – dog.*

92 *Metastatic mammary chondrosarcoma in lung – dog. H & E.*

82

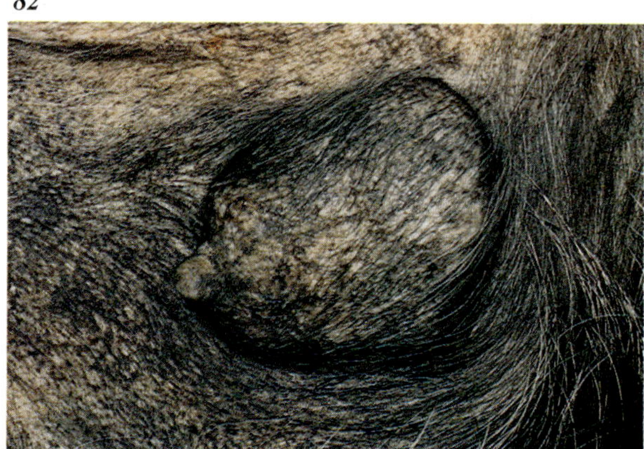

83

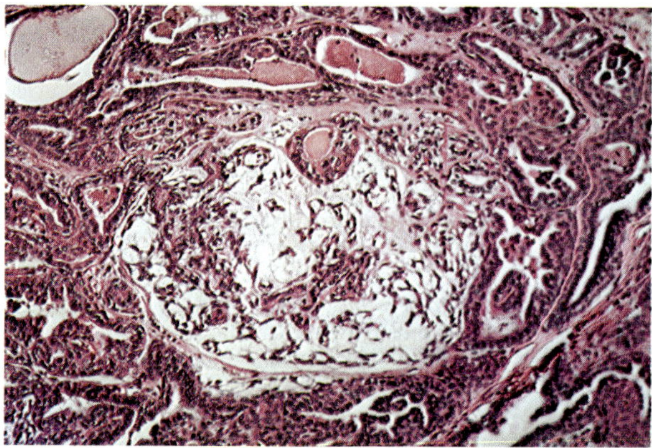

84

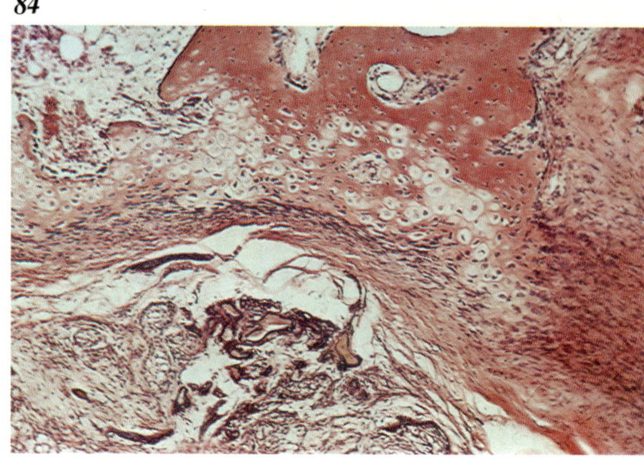

85

86

87

88

89

90

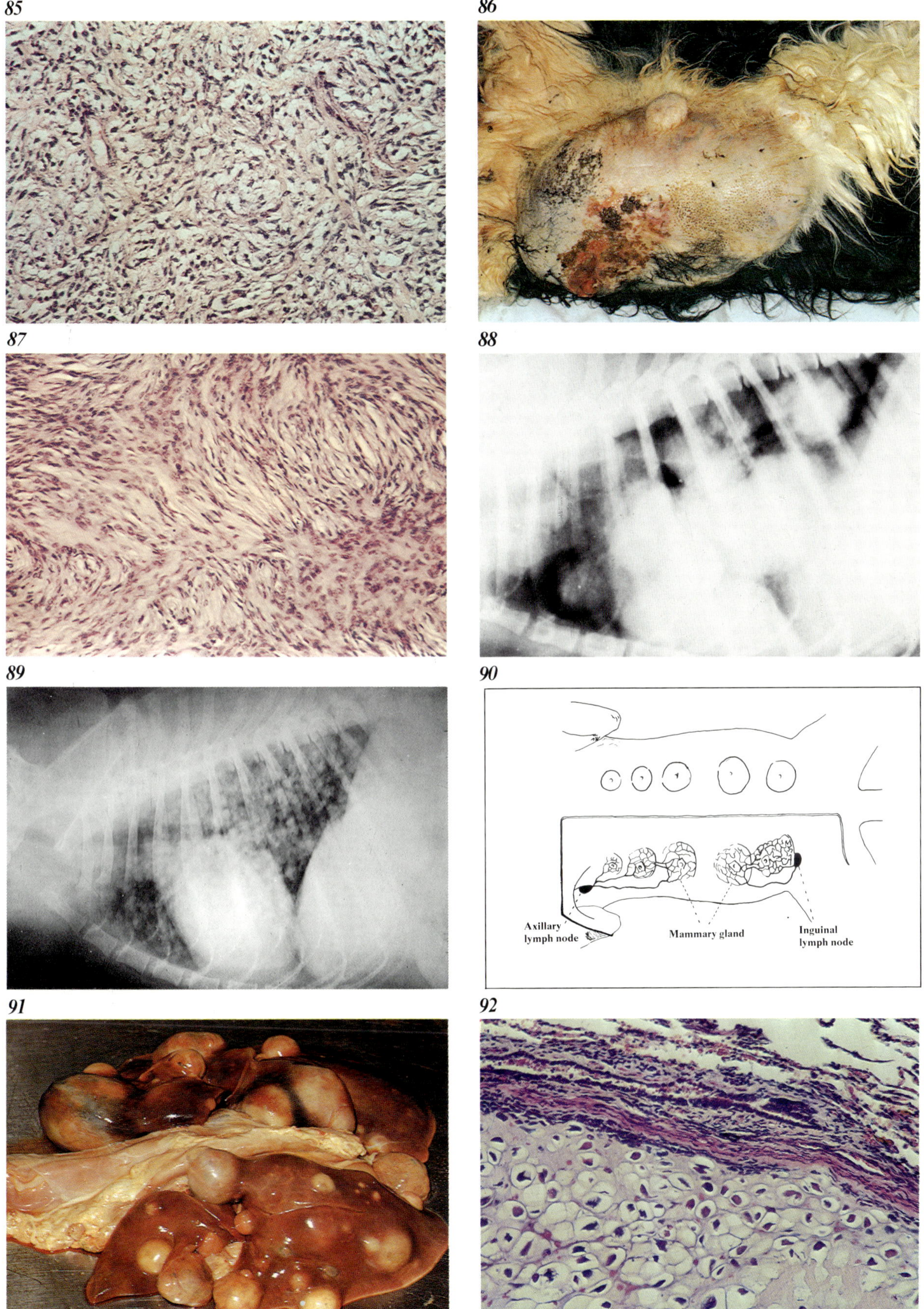

91

92

Adenomas and Carcinomas

Occurrence and gross appearance

These tumours develop from the duct or acinar epithelium of the mammary gland. They represent about 40% of the total number of mammary tumours in the dog and account for nearly all feline mammary tumours. Adenomas are much less common than carcinomas in both the dog and cat; about 95% of mammary tumours in the latter being malignant. Adenomas and carcinomas in the dog occur more frequently in the inguinal pair of glands but in the cat posterior glands are not affected more than the anterior. Mammary adenomas resemble mixed tumours, being small, circumscribed, and encapsulated, with a firm, pale, homogeneous cut surface.

Carcinomas are rapidly growing, poorly circumscribed and quickly ulcerate through the skin (***93*** *and* ***94***), which becomes secondarily infected. Adjacent glands, both on the same and opposite sides are frequently involved. The tumours are usually very firm, have a fibrous cut surface which frequently contains large areas of necrosis and have very indistinct edges.

Histological appearance

Adenomas are well circumscribed, encapsulated, and composed of closely packed acini or papillae, lined by one or more layers of cuboidal cells and filled with an eosinophilic hyaline secretion (***95***). Some adenomas in dogs are composed of large, fluid filled cysts lined by a flattened epithelium (***96***), whilst others, in both dogs and cats, have the appearance of fibroadenomas, with an abundant fibrous stroma containing foci of epithelial cells arranged as irregular tubular structures (***97***). Adenocarcinomas may be either tubular or papillary, the papillary type consisting of branching papillae lined by hyperchromatic epithelial cells arranged upon a thin fibrous septum (***98***). Low grade adenocarcinomas exhibit malignancy by invading the surrounding tissues, while the more aggressive ones show obvious vascular infiltration. Tubular adenocarcinomas are seen mainly in dogs and have a fibrous stroma which separates irregularly shaped tubules sometimes containing free, poorly differentiated cells in their centre (***99***).

Cases may be seen in which there is marked squamous metaplasia so that the tumour resembles a squamous cell carcinoma in some areas (***100***). Solid carcinomas are also common in dogs and consist of variably sized lobules of closely packed epithelial cells, with a central vesicular nucleus and indistinct cytoplasmic boundaries. Mitotic figures are conspicuous, but vascular invasion is not common (***101***). Any of these types of carcinoma may contain foci of proliferating myoepithelial cells, when they may be termed 'complex' carcinomas.

Some canine mammary carcinomas consist of poorly differentiated clumps of cells which infiltrate the surrounding tissues and vessels. The neoplastic process stimulates a prolific fibrous reaction and this type of tumour is termed an anaplastic carcinoma.

Treatment and prognosis

Simple mastectomy is indicated for clinically benign tumours and radical mastectomy for the clinically malignant tumours (***102–105***). Widespread infiltration of the dermis makes surgery difficult in many cases when response to X-irradiation is poor and local recurrence is to be expected. Some cases of the solid, rapidly growing carcinomas do respond to X-irradiation and fractionated doses up to 4,000R can be given. About 40% of all dogs which have had mammary adenocarcinomas removed surgically will eventually be destroyed because of tumour recurrence or metastasis, the majority within one year of surgery, the prognosis being linked with the degree of differentiation of the tumour. The prognosis is always poor in cats. Most animals are destroyed within a year of surgery because of pulmonary metastasis.

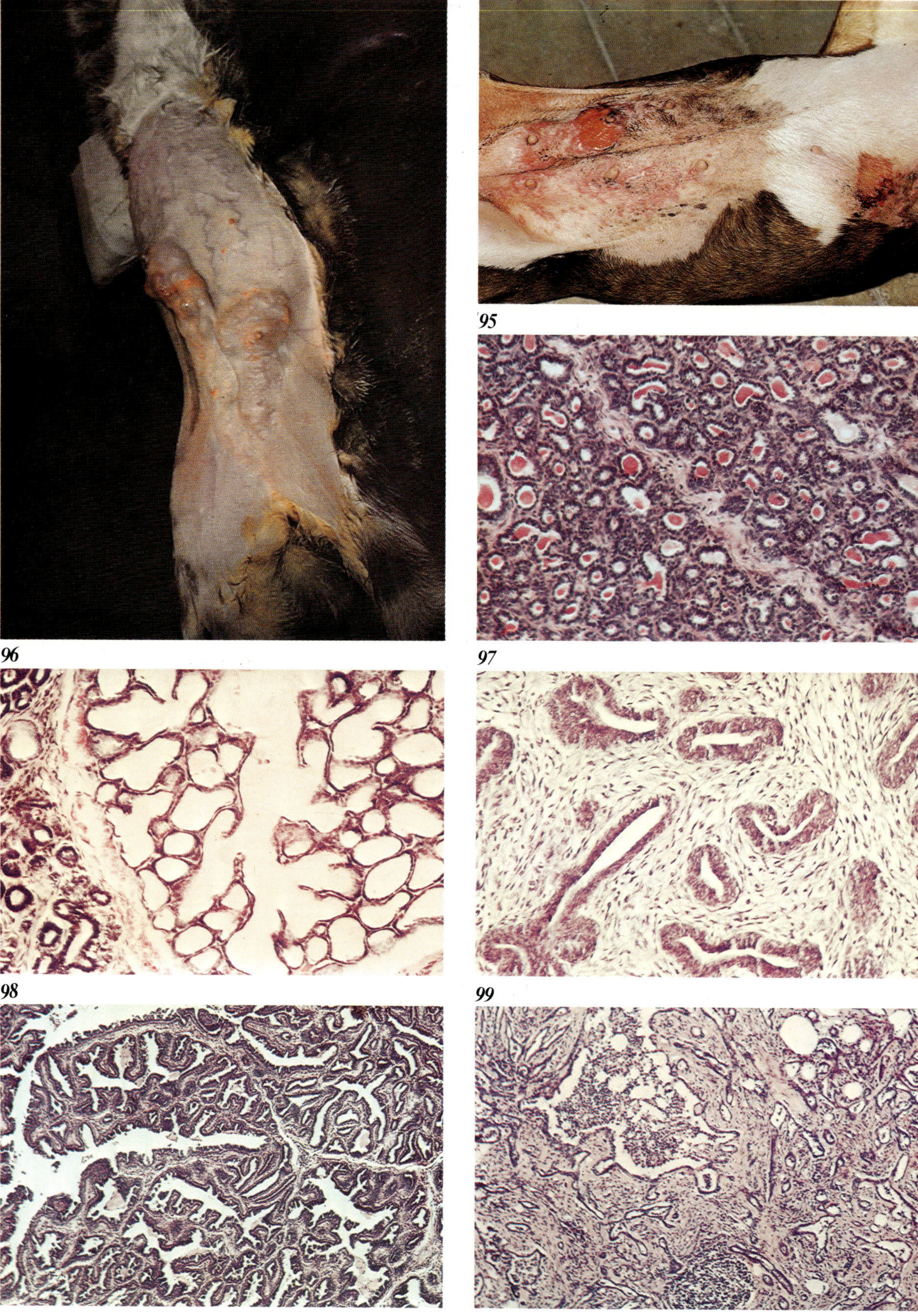
93
94
95
96
97
98
99

93 *Adenocarcinoma mammary gland – cat. The inguinal glands are* not *more favoured sites of tumour development than the pectoral glands in this species.*

94 *Tubular adenocarcinoma of mammary gland – dog. Note the ulcerative, invasive, multinodular nature of this tumour and evidence of early lymphatic spread.*

95 *Adenoma of mammary gland – dog. H & E.*

96 *Papillary cyst adenoma of mammary gland – dog. H & E.*

97 *Fibro-adenoma of mammary gland, cat. H & E.*

98 *Papillary cyst adenocarcinoma of mammary gland – cat. H & E.*

99 *Tubular adenocarcinoma of mammary gland – dog. H & E.*

100 *Adenocarcinoma of mammary gland with squamous metaplasia – dog. H & E.*

101 *Solid carcinoma of mammary gland – dog. H & E.*

102 *Mastectomy for tubular adenocarcinoma – Haemostasis.*

103 *Isolation of main vessels followed by ligation.*

104 *Completion of mastectomy.*

105 *The mastectomy wound sutured.*

100

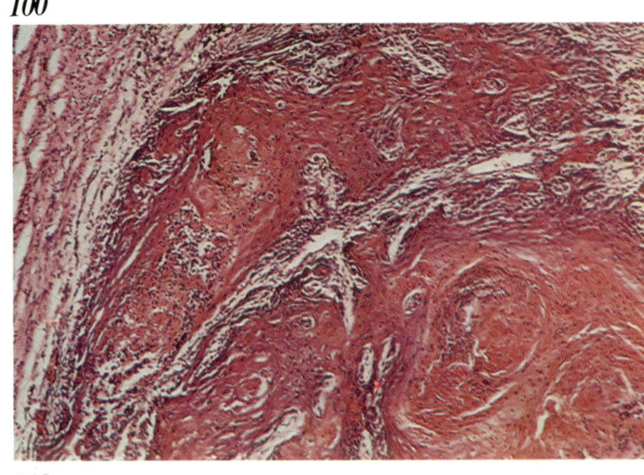

101

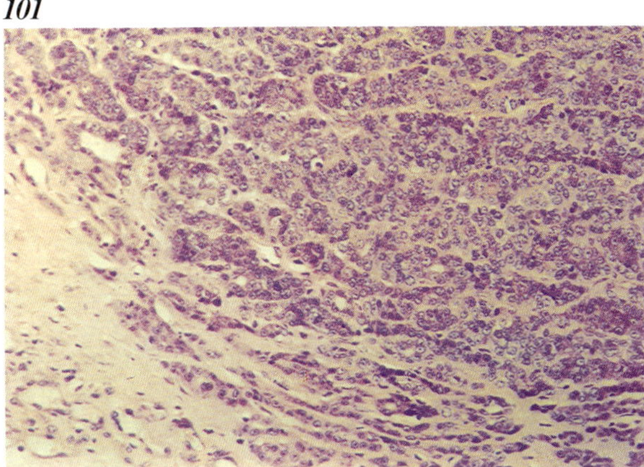

102

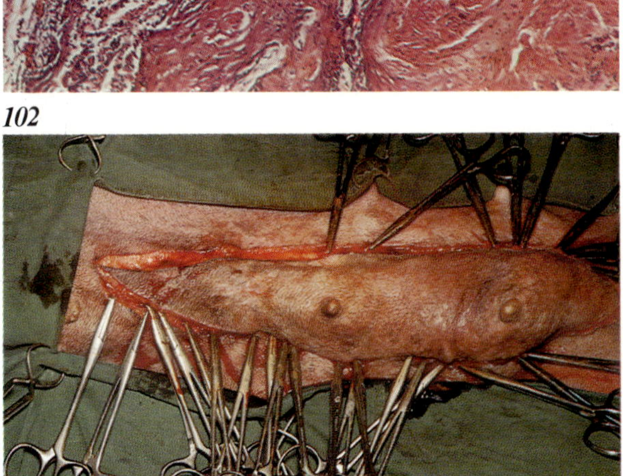

103

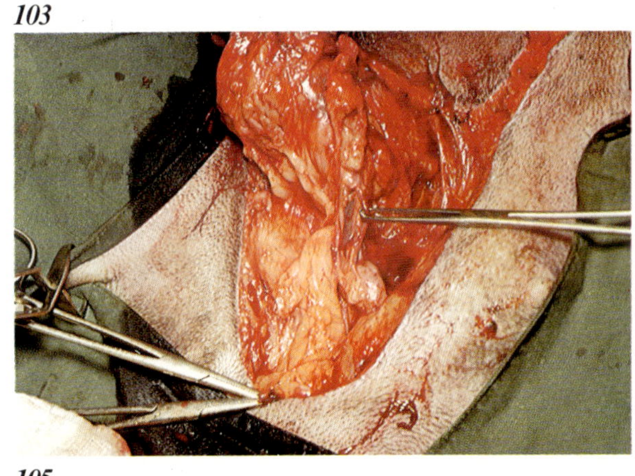

104

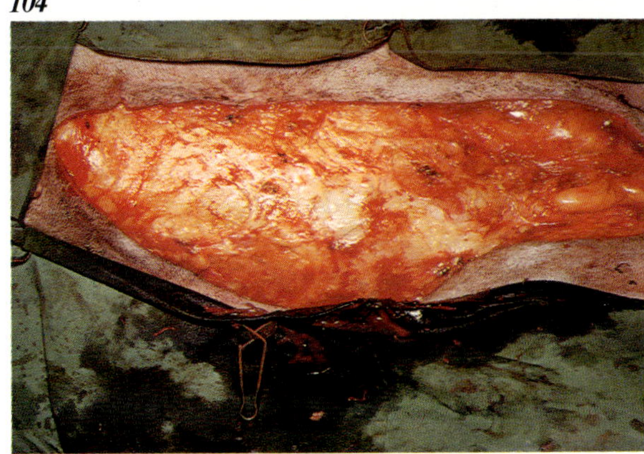

105

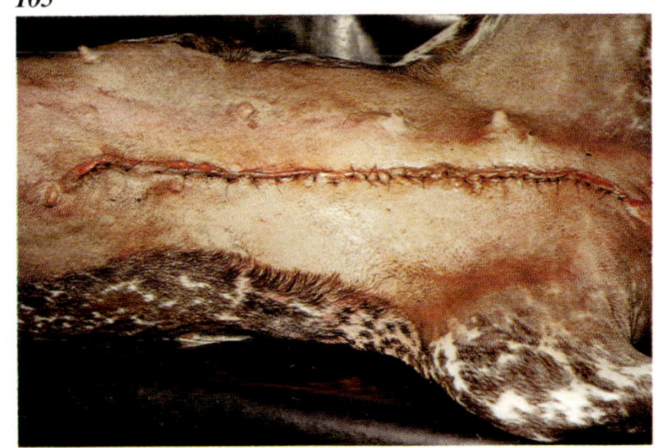

Chapter 3
The Female Genital Tract

Tumours of the female genital tract occur most commonly in the ovaries, vagina and vulva and much less frequently in the uterus and cervix.

The commonest type of ovarian neoplasm is the granulosa cell tumour. Ovarian cyst adenomas and adenocarcinomas are somewhat less common in dogs and rare in horses and cats. Dysgerminomas, which resemble seminomas morphologically, and teratomas of the ovary, are rare in all species.

In addition to the specific ovarian tissues, the connective tissue elements in the ovary may occasionally give rise to fibromas, fibrosarcomas and haemangioendotheliomas, which behave in a manner similar to these tumours in other sites.

Tumours of the vagina are common in old bitches, where they are almost always fibromas, leiomyomas, or a mixture of the two elements. Squamous cell carcinomas of the distal end of the genital tract are rare in animals, but may develop in the skin at the vulval lips in mares, where they behave in a similar manner to those in other skin sites.

The *transmissible venereal tumour*, which affects only the dog, is a naturally occurring transplantable tumour usually involving the vagina and penis. The tumour is spread from animal to animal at coitus.

Tumours of the uterus include fibromas, leiomyomas, fibroadenomas and adenocarcinomas. Chorion-epitheliomas have also been described, but are extremely rare.

In addition to the true neoplastic diseases, a number of non-neoplastic conditions may be confused with tumours. These include oestral hypertrophy of the vaginal mucosa and prolapse of the vagina in the bitch.

TUMOURS OF THE OVARY

Granulosa Cell Tumours

Occurrence and gross appearance

These are the commonest of the ovarian neoplasms and are found most frequently in mares and bitches. They are derived from the cells which line the Graafian follicles and, especially in mares, may secrete oestrogens leading to a state of continuous oestrus sometimes accompanied by the development of vicious traits. In dogs the changes are less conspicuous and the clinical signs may resemble pseudo-pregnancy, particularly in regard to the development of an enlarged abdomen.

Granulosa cell tumours can become very large before being diagnosed. They appear as roughly spherical, encapsulated, mobile masses, usually affecting only one ovary, and having a firm, lobulated, cut surface mottled by areas of haemorrhage and sometimes containing large cysts (***106***).

Histological appearance

These tumours are composed of numerous lobules of cells separated by fibrous septa. The outer zone is frequently arranged radially around the edge of the lobule (***107***), the remaining cells being closely packed. In many cases, the central area of the lobule is filled by large numbers of red blood cells or by fluid staining pink with eosin.

A relatively common variation is seen in *theca* cell tumours, which are composed entirely of sheets of large, clearly defined cells with abundant, very foamy cytoplasm, and a central, spherical nucleus (***108***). Theca cell tumours in dogs are usually small.

Treatment and prognosis

Granulosa and theca cell tumours are benign and thus surgical removal is followed by a complete cure. Removal may prove difficult in some cases because of the large size of the affected ovary.

Ovarian Adenomas and Adenocarcinomas

Occurrence and gross appearance

These tumours are seen most often in the dog but also occur in the mare and cat. They are non-functional, not associated with changes in behavioural pattern and usually manifest themselves by progressive enlargement of the abdomen. As with other ovarian tumours they may become very large before being detected and appear grossly as unilateral tumours composed of multiple, variably sized cystic structures closely packed together. The cysts are filled with a clear, yellowish fluid and lined by a whitish tissue, which even on gross examination can be seen to produce irregular, papillary ingrowths into the lumen.

Adenomas are surrounded by a thick, intact fibrous capsule while carcinomas tend to be larger and show evidence of capsular invasion. They may thus be attached closely to the serosa of the intestine or kidney, and tend to have foci of solid, whitish tissue within them, in addition to the more obviously cystic areas. Both adenomas and carcinomas can be mottled by extensive areas of haemorrhage (***109***).

Histological appearance

On microscopic examination the cysts are seen to be separated from each other by thin fibrous septa, which in the case of adenomas are lined by a well differentiated cuboidal epithelium, thrown up into numerous, branching papillary ingrowths (***110***). In adenocarcinomas the cysts tend to be smaller and to be lined by less well differentiated cells which round up to form small rosettes within the lumen (***111***). There is obvious invasion of the stroma and capsule with extension into the surrounding tissues. The most malignant tumours tend to lose their cystic structure almost entirely, and consist of solid sheets of closely packed, poorly differentiated epithelial cells, amongst which mitotic figures are very common (***112***).

106

107

108

109

110

111

112

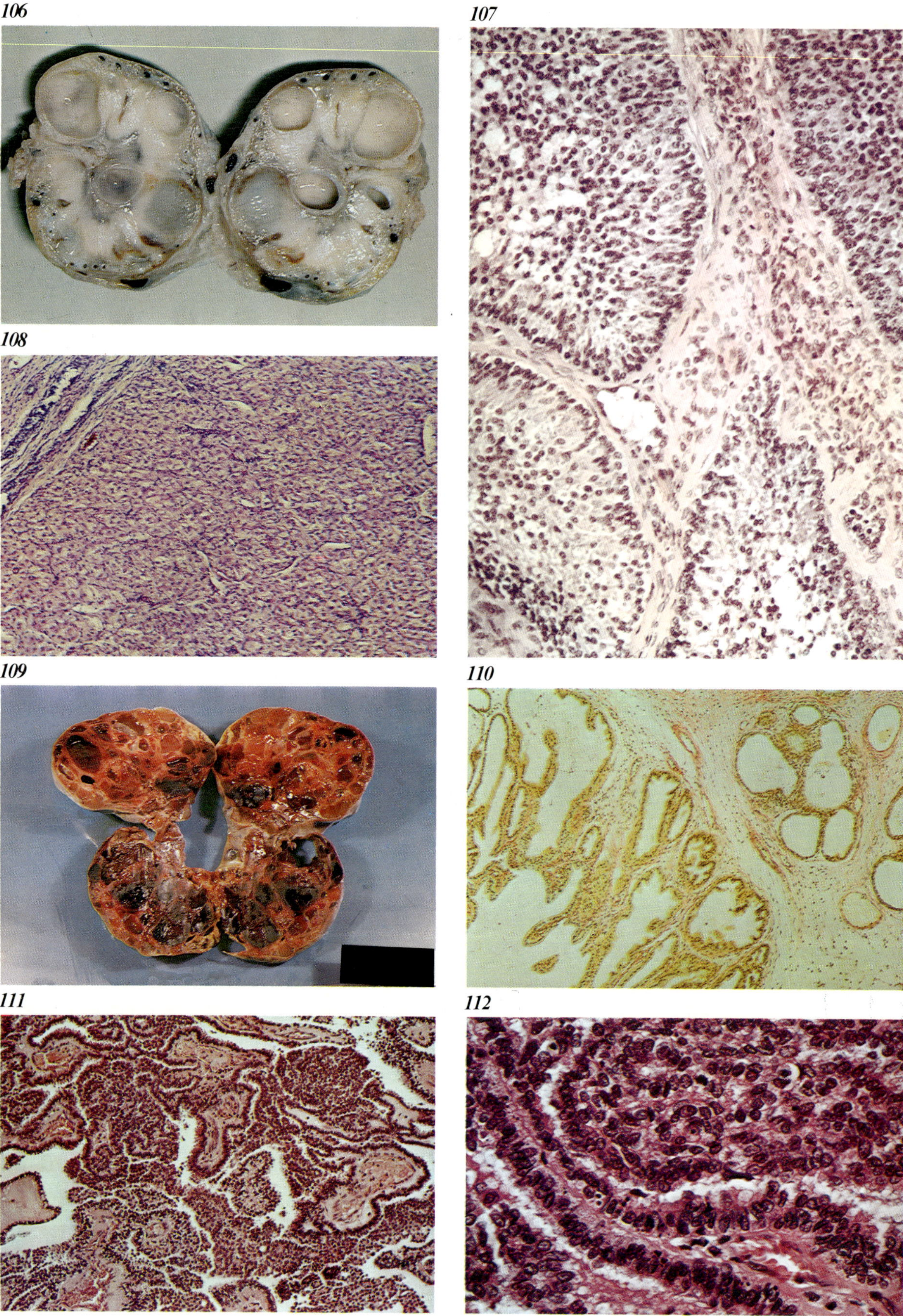

106 *Granulosa cell tumour – mare. Both ovaries were similarly affected.*

107 *Granulosa cell tumour – mare. Note the palisading of cells at the periphery of each focus. H & E.*

108 *Theca cell tumour – dog. H & E.*

109 *Ovarian adenoma – dog. Many of the cysts contain blood.*

110 *Ovarian adenoma – dog. Van Gieson.*

111 *Ovarian adenocarcinoma – dog. H & E.*

112 *Poorly differentiated ovarian adenocarcinoma – dog. H & E.*

Aetiology

Many cases of cystic ovarian disease show areas resembling early adenomatous change, and this suggests a possible hormonal aetiology.

Treatment and prognosis

Adenomas can become very large before they are diagnosed, but provided the animal survives the immediate post surgical period, skilled excision is followed by a complete cure. The prognosis following removal of an ovarian carcinoma must always be guarded. Many of these tumours cannot be completely excised because they are adherent to surrounding structures so that local recurrence and metastasis following surgery are to be expected. The common mode of spread is intra-abdominal, with multiple small, firm whitish tumours appearing on the parietal and visceral peritoneum. Spread by the haematogenous route also occurs to produce metastases in the liver and lungs.

Cystic Ovarian Disease

Occurrence and gross appearance

This condition, which sometimes resembles ovarian neoplasia, and which may be a pre-neoplastic lesion, can occur in all three species, but is seen most often in dogs, where it is relatively common in middle-aged or older bitches. It usually affects both ovaries, although unequally, and tends to be seen in animals with a history of irregular oestrus cycles. The cysts, which develop from Graafian follicles, occur frequently in the ovaries of bitches with pyometra (***113***), although a causal relationship has not been established. The degree of cystic change is very variable, some affected ovaries being completely replaced by a closely packed mass of turgid, thin walled cysts filled with a clear watery fluid (***114***), while in others the ovarian cortex contains a few large, cystic structures.

In the mare cystic ovaries frequently give rise to behavioural changes including permanent oestrus.

Histological appearance

The cysts are well differentiated and lined by a single layer of flattened cuboidal epithelial cells showing some tendency towards forming papillary ingrowths (***115***). In some cases, areas resembling true adenomas are seen, making it difficult to distinguish the two conditions.

Aetiology
Hormonal treatment, especially progesterone, may predispose to cystic ovarian disease in bitches.

Treatment and prognosis
The lesions are well encapsulated and surgical excision of both ovaries is generally simple. The condition is a common incidental post mortem finding in the bitch and its clinical significance is uncertain in this species.

TUMOURS OF THE UTERUS, CERVIX AND VAGINA

Fibromas and Fibrosarcomas

Occurrence and gross appearance
Fibrosarcomas of the female genital tract are rare in all three species, but fibromas are common in old, non-spayed bitches. They occur most frequently in the vagina, where they may be numerous but may also be found in the cervix or uterine wall. They are slowly growing tumours which either appear at the vulval opening accompanied by a haemorrhagic vaginal discharge, or present as a firm, spherical mass in the perineum (***116***), which causes difficulty in defaecation. They are well circumscribed, spherical, often pedunculated tumours, covered by a thin epithelium which usually ulcerates and becomes infected. The cut surface is homogeneous, whitish in colour, fibrous in consistency (***117***) and only rarely contains areas of haemorrhage and necrosis.

Histological appearance
Some vaginal and uterine fibromas have a very similar appearance to those previously described in the skin (***118***), but many have an obvious and sometimes predominant smooth muscle component. The smooth muscle appears as parallel bundles of well differentiated, elongated cells forming syncytia, distributed in a random fashion within the fibrous tissue. Leiomyomas, composed entirely of smooth muscle, are also seen (***119***).

Treatment and prognosis
Surgical removal of vaginal tumours may be performed following episiotomy but those in the cervix and uterus are accessible only following laparotomy. The prognosis after excision is favourable with most animals showing no evidence of tumour regrowth.

---

113 *Cystic ovary in a bitch with pyometra. Uterine fibromas are also present.*

114 *Cystic ovary – dog. Note the multiple, thin-walled, turgid cysts.*

115 *Cystic ovary – dog. H & E.*

116 *Fibroma of vagina in a 10-year-old bitch. These tumours often present as a firm, mobile swelling in the perineum.*

117 *Cut surface of canine vaginal fibroma.*

118 *Vaginal fibroma. H & E.*

119 *Vaginal leiomyoma. H & E.*

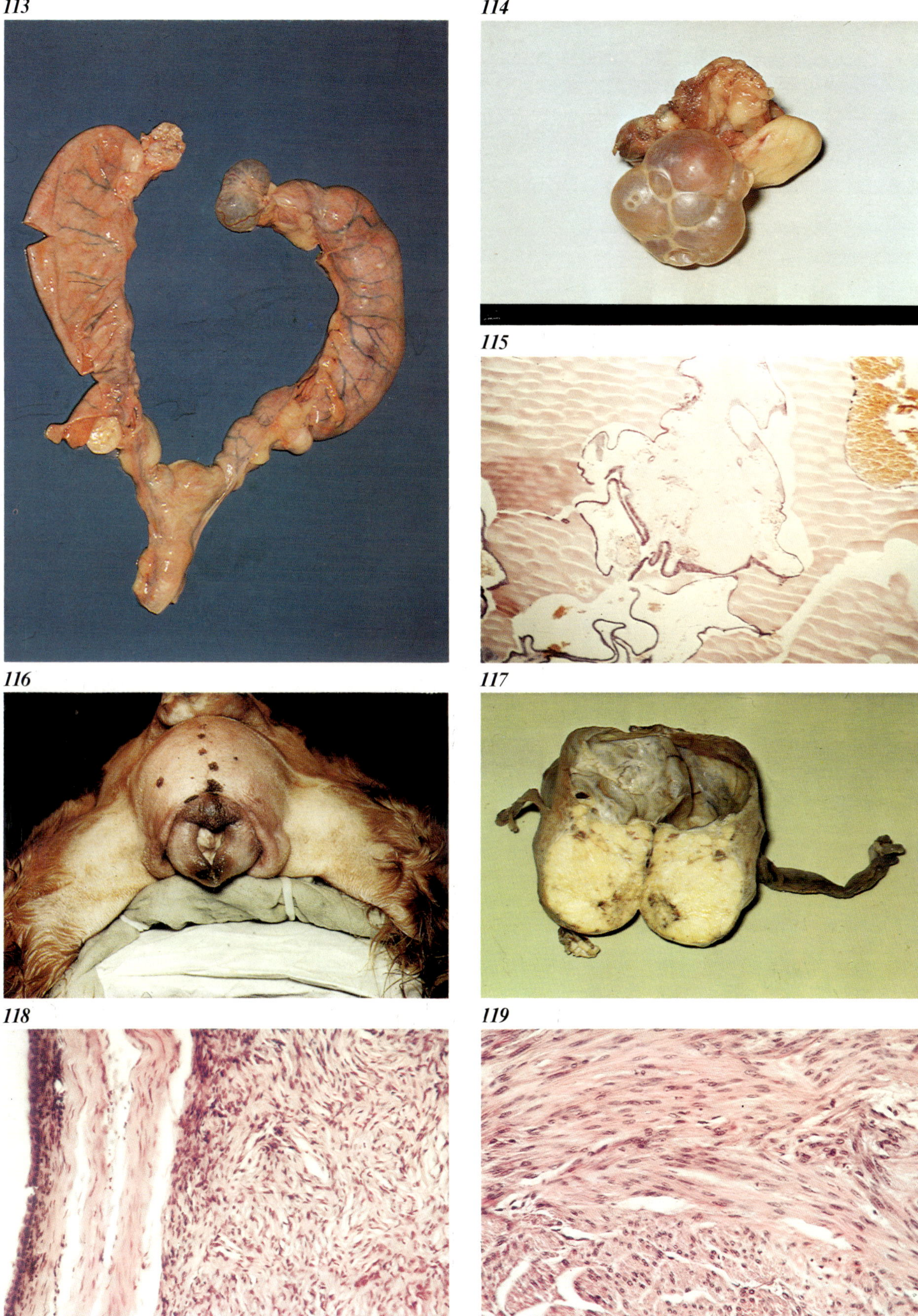
113
114
115
116
117
118
119

Occasionally tumours are so large or numerous when the animal is first seen that surgery cannot be attempted. It has been suggested that ovaro-hysterectomy will reduce the growth of vaginal fibromas, but at present there are too few controlled clinical observations to substantiate this.

Adenomas and Adenocarcinomas

Occurrence and gross appearance

Epithelial tumours of the female genital tract are very rare in the horse, dog and cat. They are seen most frequently in the uterus of the dog, in which benign tumours are more common than malignant.

Adenomas can be very large, are usually single, and grow into the lumen of the uterus. They are well circumscribed, pedunculated, firm in consistency and covered by an intact mucosa (***120***). The cut surface is pale yellowish in colour and variably sized cysts, filled with a clear, yellowish fluid, may be present.

Carcinomas appear in the uterus or vagina as flattened, poorly circumscribed tumours invading the wall of the organ and ulcerating through the mucosa. They have a firm, whitish homogeneous cut surface, which does not contain macroscopic cysts.

Histological appearance

Most adenomas of the genital tract are composed of a very dense stroma of mature collagen which contains a number of well differentiated acinar structures, lined by a single layer of epithelial cells and frequently containing secretion (***121***). Carcinomas are diffusely invasive and consist of numerous, closely packed and irregularly shaped acini, the lining cells of which are thrown into papillary ingrowths protruding into the lumen (***122***). Squamous cell carcinomas of the cervix are rare.

Treatment and prognosis

Ovaro-hysterectomy in the bitch usually results in a complete cure, even in animals with histologically malignant tumours.

Transmissible Venereal Tumour

Occurrence and gross appearance

This tumour occurs only in the dog, where it is widely distributed throughout the world, occurring more commonly in tropical or sub-tropical areas. It is common in parts of Africa, Malaysia, and the Carribean, but is seen, infrequently, in Northern and Western Europe. Lesions are usually confined to the mucous membrane of the penis and vagina, but can occasionally be found in the mouth or lips. The most common clinical manifestation is a bloodstained discharge from the prepuce or vulva, and in females the tumour may protrude from the lips of the vulva where it appears as a soft, friable, pinkish mass (***123***), with an ulcerated and infected surface. In the male the penis must usually be exposed manually before the tumour becomes visible. The appearance is of a multinodular, invasive and poorly circumscribed tumour, closely attached to the penis and prepuce (***124***), and having a pink, fleshy cut surface.

Histological appearance

Tumours from different animals all have a very similar morphology, being composed of a closely packed sheet of large cells, with eosinophilic cytoplasm apparent , and a rather pale staining nucleus. Cytoplasmic boundaries are indistinct, mitotic figures are common, and the cells are not arranged in any obvious architectural pattern (***125***). In some cases small clumps of cells are surrounded by fine reticulin fibres and it has been suggested that this tumour is derived from reticulum cells.

Aetiology

It appears that in spite of its name, this tumour is transplantable rather than transmissible, living cells being transferred from one animal to another at coitus. Studies on tumours from animals in widely different parts of the world have revealed all the cells to contain a similar number (59 ± 5) of chromosomes, instead of the normal 78. Attempts at transmission using cell-free extracts have failed and immunological studies indicate that the tumour is unlikely to be of viral origin.

Treatment and prognosis

A small percentage of dogs with transmissible venereal tumours exhibit spontaneous regression of the neoplasm without treatment, following which they are unlikely to develop further tumours. A few animals exhibit metastases, usually to the inguinal lymph nodes, but occasionally to more distant organs, while many have to be destroyed because of the large size of the primary tumour. Complete surgical removal is often very difficult because of the diffuse nature of the tumour, and local recurrence is common. The tumour is, however, radiosensitive and complete and permanent regression occurs after fractionated doses up to 3,000R X-irradiation. Results using autogenous vaccines produced from killed tumour cells have usually been disappointing.

120 *Cyst-adenoma. Uterus of bitch.*

121 *Adenoma of uterus – dog. H & E.*

122 *Papillary adenocarcinoma of uterus – dog. H & E.*

123 *Transmissible venereal tumour of vagina appearing at the vulva of a two-year-old African 'Bush' dog.*

124 *Transmissible venereal tumour of penis and prepuce.*

125 *Transmissible venereal tumour. Note the poorly differentiated nature of the tumour and its malignant histological appearance. H & E.*

120

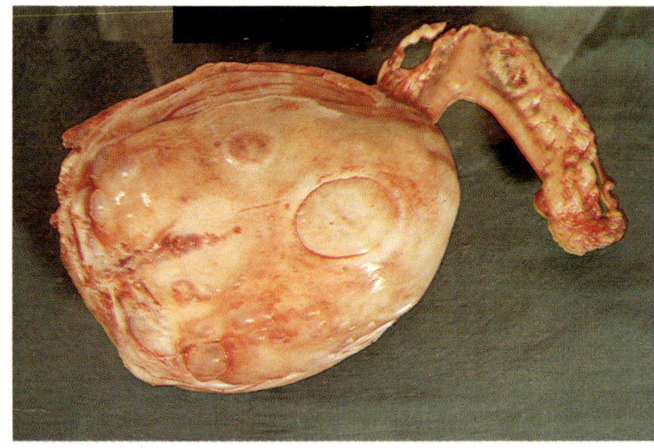

121

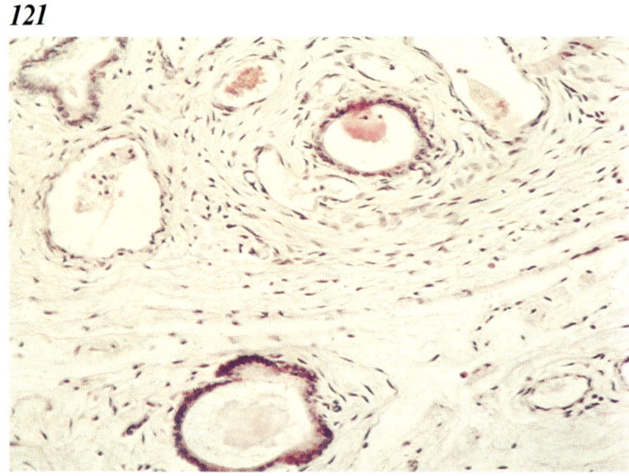

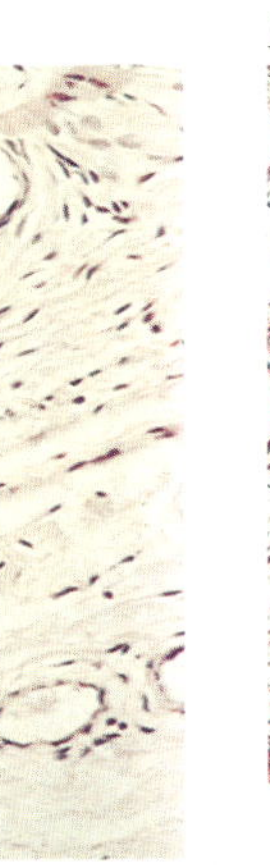

122

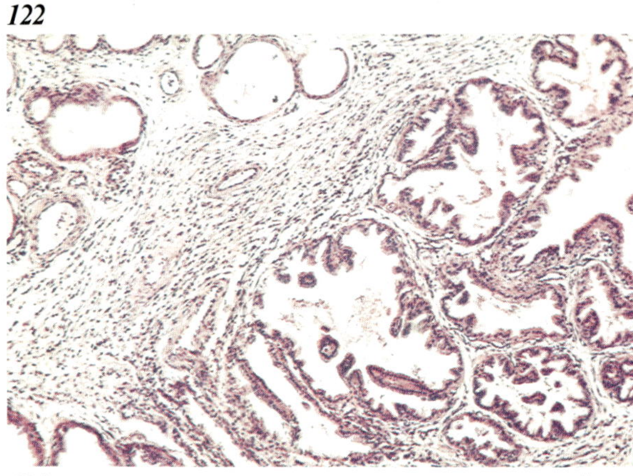

123

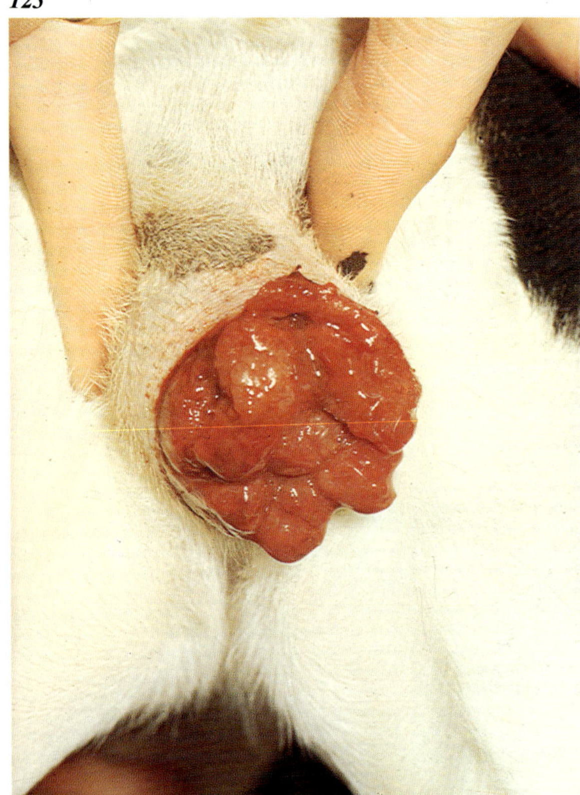

124

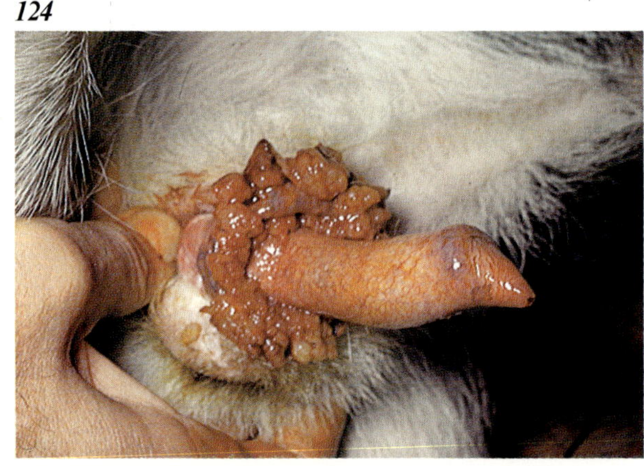

125

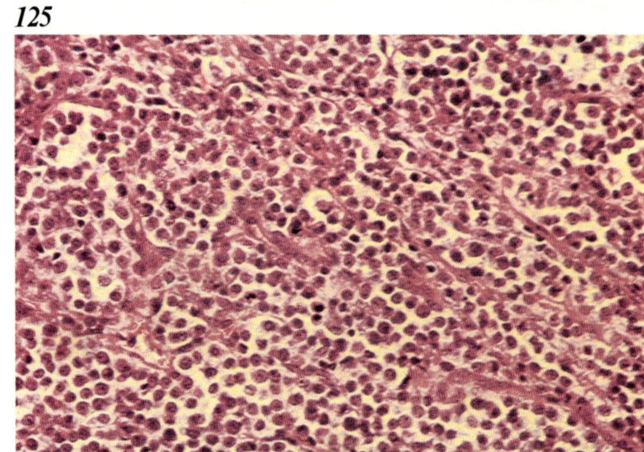

NON-NEOPLASTIC TUMOUR-LIKE LESIONS

Oestral Hypertrophy of the Vagina

Occurrence and gross appearance

Although this condition is not neoplastic, it is frequently confused with vaginal neoplasia and must be distinguished from it. The condition is seen only in dogs, and appears to be especially common in Boxers and Labrador Retrievers. It usually manifests itself in young adults a few days after the beginning of the first or second oestrus period as a soft, rubbery, pinkish mass of tissue which protrudes from the lips of the vulva. It arises from the floor of the vagina, and usually enlarges very rapidly to reach maximum size in a few days (*126*).

Histological appearance

This is quite typical, the mass consisting of a very loose oedematous stroma covered by an intact mucosa (*127*).

Aetiology

The immediate cause is hormonal, but it is possible that certain strains of dog are more likely to develop the condition, indicating a genetic basis.

Treatment and prognosis

The prognosis should always be favourable since the hypertrophied tissue returns to normal at the end of oestrus. The condition may prove troublesome however since severe lesions can interfere with mating. Surgical removal is possible but may only be partially successful, and because of the possible genetic factors the most satisfactory method of treatment is ovaro-hysterectomy. Following this procedure, a complete cure is ensured.

126 *Oestral hypertrophy of the vagina in a young Boxer bitch.*

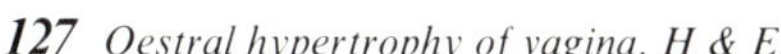

127 *Oestral hypertrophy of vagina. H & E.*

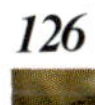

126

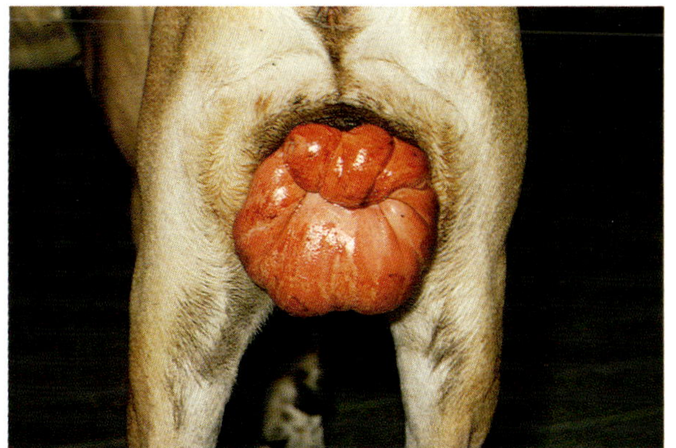

127

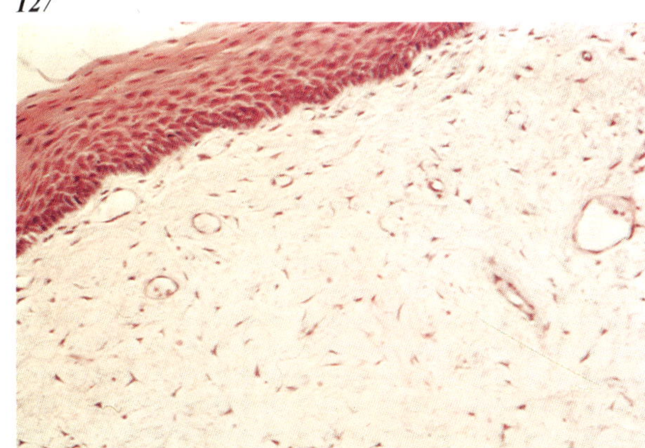

Chapter 4
The Male Genital Tract

Testicular tumours are seen commonly in the dog, but are very rare in the other two species, perhaps because so many male cats and horses are castrated early in life.

In the dog the commonest type is the Leydig (*interstitial*) cell tumour, about 20 % of middle-aged and older dogs having small, frequently bilateral lesions of this type in their testes. Most of these tumours are clinically inapparent and are detected incidentally on post mortem examination. Sertoli cell tumours are not uncommon while seminomas are seen somewhat less frequently.

Connective tissue tumours are very rare in the testes themselves, but neoplasms arising in the scrotal skin may sometimes invade the testis. Teratomas, found in the testes of young adult stallions, occur more frequently in cryptorchid animals and are rare.

A number of conditions which affect the testis may be confused with neoplasms and of these bacterial orchitis and scrotal hernia are by far the most important.

Benign cystic degeneration and hyperplasia are common changes seen in the prostate of old dogs and can be confused with neoplasms. True tumours are rare, but when they do occur are usually malignant.

Tumours affecting the prepuce and penis have been described elsewhere.

Leydig Cell Tumours (Interstitial Adenomas)

Occurrence and gross appearance

This is the commonest testicular tumour in dogs, but is rare in the other species. It occurs in both descended and cryptorchid testes and is frequently bilateral. Middle-aged or older dogs are usually affected, and many tumours of this type are not clinically apparent. Tumours which are found incidentally at post mortem are usually only 1–2cm in diameter and are seen within the substance of the testis. They are very well circumscribed and have a reddish-yellow, bulging, homogeneous cut surface (***128***).

The larger, clinically apparent tumours are very often cystic, and may be up to 5–6cm in diameter. They consist of a single, thick walled cyst filled with a colourless fluid and lined by yellowish, homogeneous tissue surrounded by a dense fibrous capsule. There is frequently a remnant of the testis at one edge of the tumour.

Histological appearance

The Leydig cell tumour is well encapsulated and clearly demarcated from surrounding tissues. It consists of large epithelial cells with a central, spherical nucleus and abundant eosinophilic cytoplasm, the cells being arranged as solid sheets, cords or small acini. Sometimes the cells are seen lining blood-filled spaces, and may be seen arranged as rosettes around small blood vessels (*129*). Mitotic figures are rare.

Treatment and prognosis
Following castration the prognosis is good as malignancy is extremely rare. Leydig cell tumours are not known to produce functional hormone secretions and the behaviour of the affected dog is not altered.

Sertoli (Sustentacular) Cell Tumours

Occurrence and gross appearance
These tumours are seen almost exclusively in older dogs and are the testicular tumours which most commonly give rise to clinical signs. They occur more often in the right testis than the left and are frequent in cryptorchid testes.

They are relatively slow growing, non-invasive, painless tumours which may become very large. The cut surface is pale in colour, and contains numerous lobules of raised white tissue (*128*). Intra-abdominal tumours tend to be more irregular in shape, frequently appearing as multinodular masses, but they also have a firm, pale cut surface.

Some Sertoli cell tumours secrete oestrogens which lead to very characteristic changes of feminisation in the affected animal, the dog becoming sexually attractive to other males. Often there is enlargement of the nipples, bilateral alopecia with pigmentation of the skin, enlargement of the prepuce and atrophy of the non-tumorous testis (*130–132*). The prostate may also become enlarged due to squamous metaplasia (*133*).

Histological appearance
In the early case the tubules are relatively normal in size but spermatogenesis is in abeyance and the tubules become lined by well oriented, tall, columnar cells with foamy, pale-staining cytoplasm and an oval, hyperchromatic nucleus (*134*). As the disease progresses the interstitial collagen becomes much more abundant, and obliterates many tubules, those which remain becoming dilated and lined by many layers of irregularly shaped cells. In most tubules a small central lumen is preserved and the basal layer of cells retains its well orientated nature, with obvious 'palisading' of the nuclei (*135*). Mitotic figures may be seen in the cells, but vascular invasion is unusual.

Treatment and prognosis
Since the tunica vaginalis remains intact surgical excision is straightforward, following which signs of feminisation and alopecia disappear spontaneously within about four months. In a minority of cases metastases develop in the iliac lymph nodes (*136*), but the prognosis for most animals with intrascrotal tumours is favourable.

In dogs with intra-abdominal tumours the prognosis is more guarded since trans-abdominal spread, especially to the posterior pole of the ipsilateral kidney, is common.

Seminomas

Occurrence and gross appearance
Seminomas are less common than Sertoli cell tumours. They occur in middle-aged or

128 *Testicular tumours in the dog. Left, Leydig cell tumour. Right, Sertoli cell tumour.*

129 *Leydig cell tumour. The cells often form rosettes around blood vessels. H & E.*

130 *Gynecomastia and oedema of the sheath in a Boxer with a functional Sertoli cell tumour.*

131 *Alopecia and hyperpigmentation of the skin of the ventral abdomen due to a functional Sertoli cell tumour.*

132 *Sertoli cell tumour in left testis with atrophy of the right testis.*

133 *Squamous metaplasia of the prostate in a dog with a Sertoli cell tumour. H & E.*

134 *Early Sertoli cell tumour – dog. Spermatogenesis is in abeyance and the tubules are lined by well oriented columnar cells with pale staining foamy cytoplasm. H & E.*

135 *Advanced Sertoli cell tumour – dog. Many tubules have been replaced by a dense fibrous stroma. Van Gieson.*

136 *Metastasis to iliac lymph nodes from a Sertoli cell tumour.*

137 *Seminoma in right testis. The testis has not fully descended and is in the inguinal canal.*

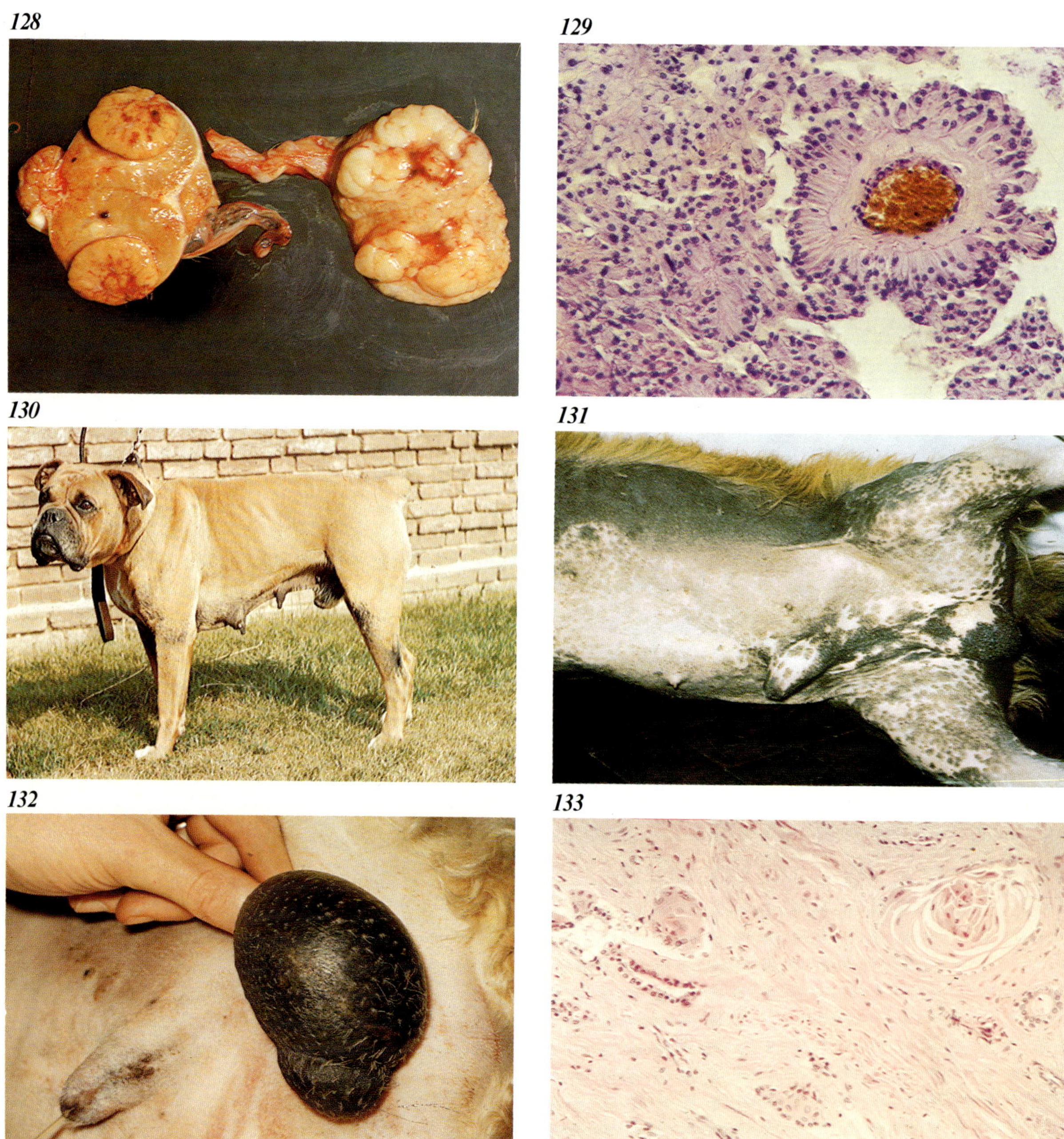

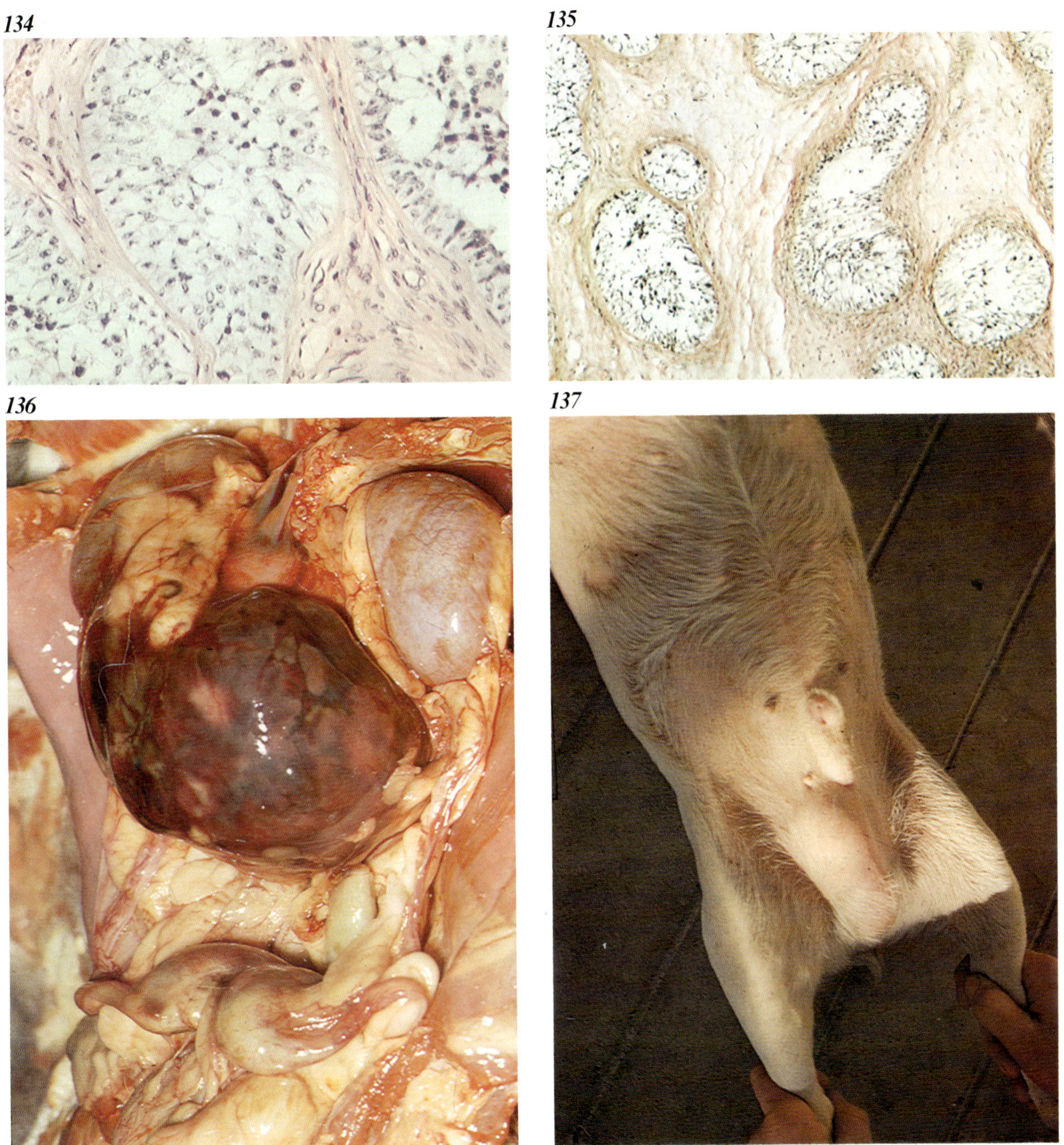

134 135

136 137

older dogs and are more frequent in the cryptorchid than the normal testis (*137*). While tending to replace the entire structure of the testis they do not usually destroy the capsule, and are thus easy to remove surgically, although intra-abdominal tumours may become very large before advice is sought. They have a friable yellowish-white cut surface frequently mottled by areas of necrosis and haemorrhage. There is no evidence that seminomas produce functional hormones.

Histological appearance

In early cases the tumour cells are confined within the seminiferous tubules but the basement membranes are rapidly lost and the typical appearance is of a homogeneous sheet of large, closely packed cells which have completely replaced the normal testicular structure. The cells are round or polygonal and have a central, roughly spherical, hyperchromatic nucleus and a variable but usually abundant amount of eosinophilic cytoplasm. The cells are not arranged in any defined architectural pattern, and do not produce an obvious intercellular matrix. Mitotic figures are seen commonly and the tumour has a very malignant appearance (***138***).

Treatment and prognosis

Following castration the prognosis is usually favourable although a small number of tumours metastasise to the iliac lymph nodes and occasionally the lungs. The prognosis for dogs with intra-abdominal tumours is more guarded however as the primary tumour tends to be larger when first diagnosed, and trans-abdominal spread, especially to the kidneys and omentum, is not uncommon.

Teratomas

These tumours appear as roughly spherical, well defined masses with a heterogeneous cut surface in the testis or ovary, especially in young horses, although they may rarely appear in the ovary of dogs. They contain solid areas and variably sized cystic structures which may contain hairs or teeth (***139***), and histologically are seen to consist of a variety of tissues not normally arranged in any definite form.

Following surgical excision the prognosis is favourable although occasionally one of the constituents will undergo malignant transformation and produce distant metastases.

Prostatic Carcinomas

Occurrence and gross appearance

Carcinoma of the prostate is rare in the dog and not recorded in the cat or horse. When the prostate is intra-pelvic a hard, irregular, knobbly mass can be palpated per rectum. The capsule is invaded early so that the prostate becomes adherent to the surrounding tissues, invading particularly the serosa of the bladder, especially near its neck.

Histological appearance

Highly invasive, with an abundant fibrous stroma containing irregular acinar or papillary structures, lined by one or more layers of hyperchromatic epithelial cells (***140***). Rapidly growing tumours may consist of a solid sheet of undifferentiated cells.

Treatment and prognosis

The prognosis is poor as surgical excision is extremely difficult and regional lymph node and visceral metastasis is common. Castration followed by a subcutaneous implant of stilboestrol (15–30mg) may lead to temporary regression.

NON-NEOPLASTIC TUMOUR-LIKE LESIONS

Benign Hyperplasia of the Prostate

Occurrence and gross appearance

Benign prostate hyperplasia occurs mainly in the dog and is often manifested clinically by difficulty in defaecation or urination. The grossly enlarged gland may or may not be palpable per rectum but radiographic examination of the abdominal cavity, especially with the aid of a pneumocystogram (***141***), can often help in locating the position of the prostate more accurately. Direct examination of the affected organ reveals it to be roughly bilaterally symmetrical (***142***), with a very firm, granular, pale cut surface sometimes containing small, fluid filled cysts (***143***).

Histological appearance

Cases uncomplicated by secondary infection show loss of the normal acini which are replaced by large, irregularly shaped cystic structures lined by a single layer of well differentiated columnar cells. The lining membrane is characteristically thrown up into numerous papillae which branch within the cyst lumen (***144***). Bundles of smooth muscle and collagen are present in the stroma and as the condition progresses the amount of collagen increases. If secondary infection supervenes large areas of necrosis and haemorrhage develop.

Aetiology

The initial glandular hyperplasia is probably due to hormonal stimulation but the exact cause is obscure.

Treatment and prognosis

Surgical removal of the pathological canine prostate is not easy and usually results in incontinence. The best form of treatment in those cases where secondary infection is not severe is castration. Castration plus the administration of anti-testosterone drugs such as delmadinone acetate, 1–1.5mg/kg/day for eight days has also been advocated. Stilboestrol, 15–30mg as a subcutaneous implant, has been used to reduce the size of the prostate but prolonged administration may lead to secondary enlargement due to squamous metaplasia.

If secondary infection is severe, the prognosis must always be poor, antibiotic therapy apparently being of little value in these cases.

138 *Seminoma – dog. The normal tubular architecture has been lost and replaced by a homogeneous sheet of actively proliferating cells. H & E.*

139 *Teratoma testicle – horse. Note the presence of hair and teeth.*

140 *Prostatic adenocarcinoma – dog. H & E.*

141 *Pneumocystogram benign prostatic hyperplasia – dog. The prostate is symmetrically enlarged and is outside the pelvic canal.*

138

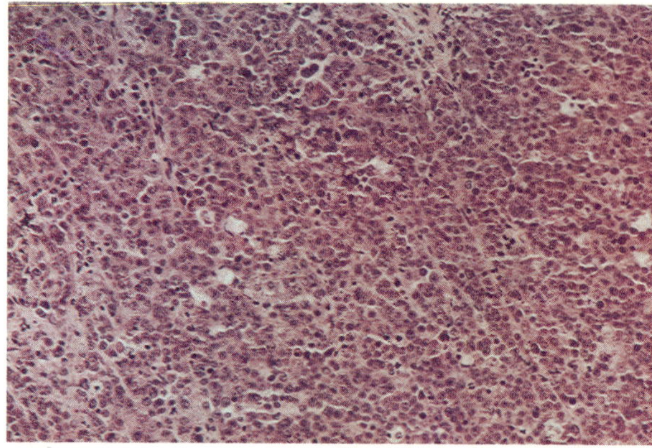

139

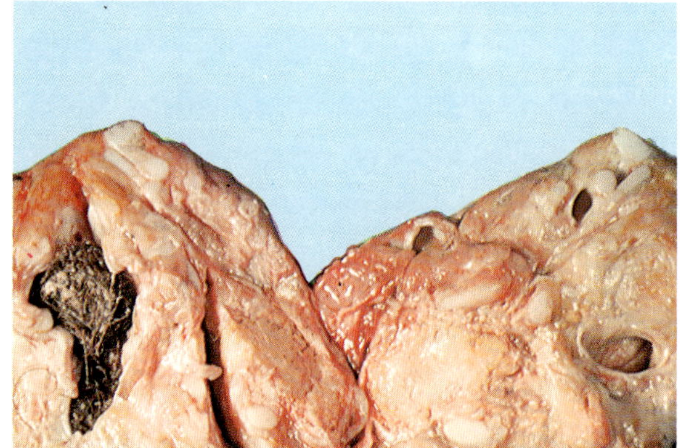

140

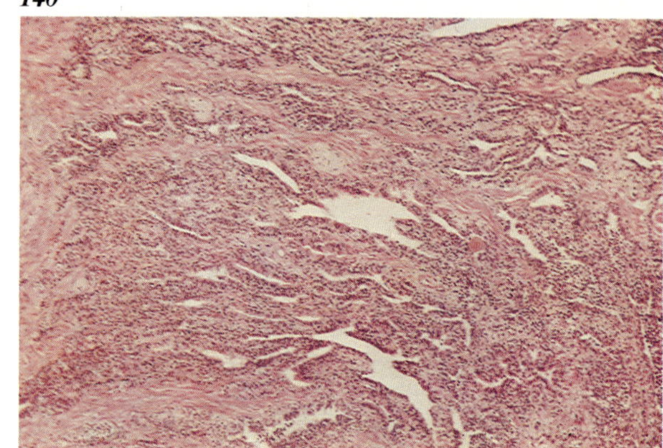

141

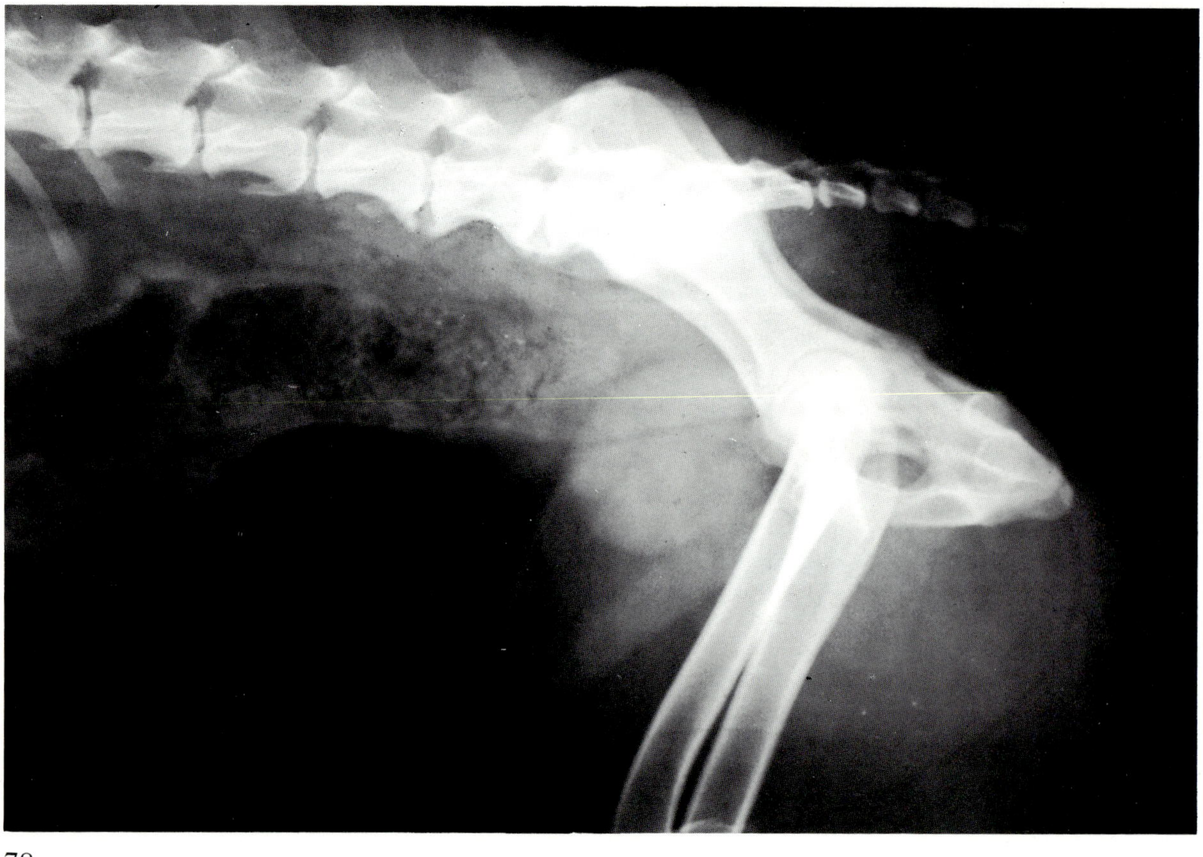

142

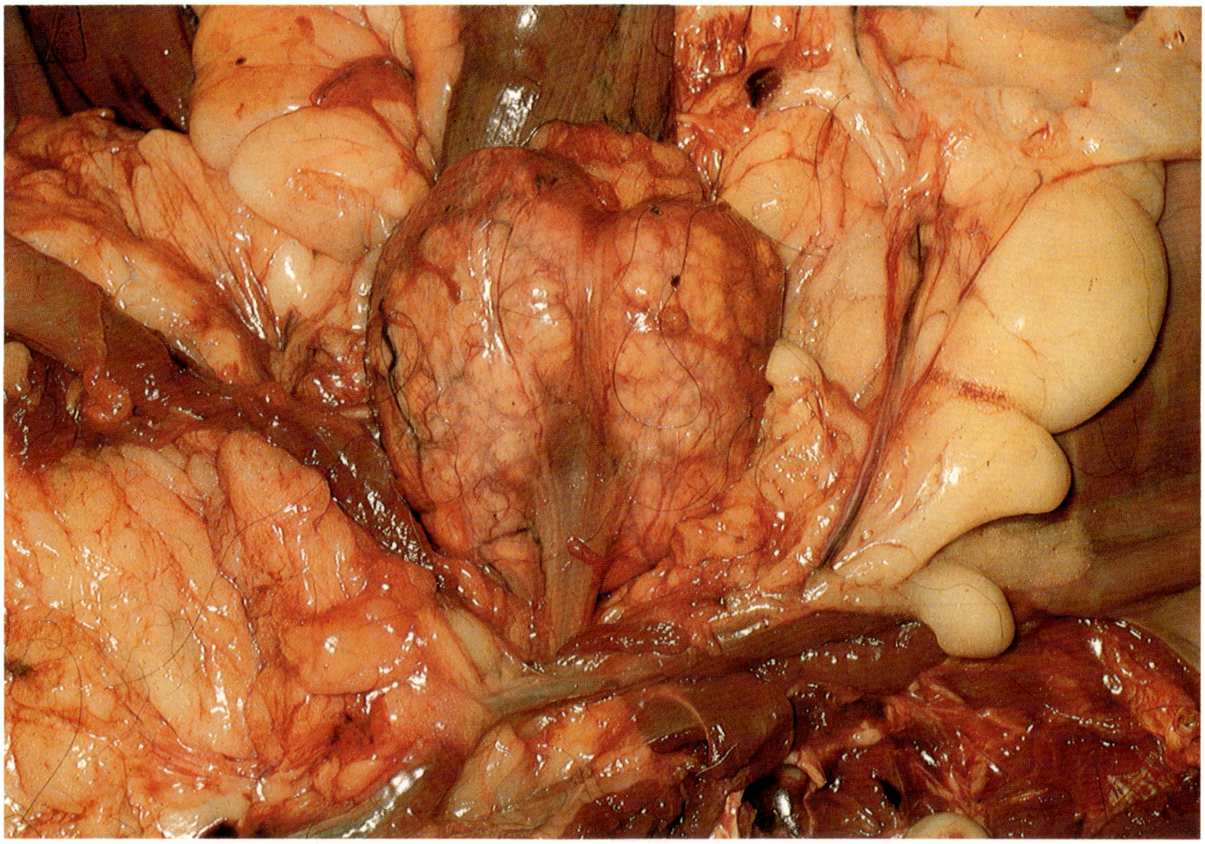

143

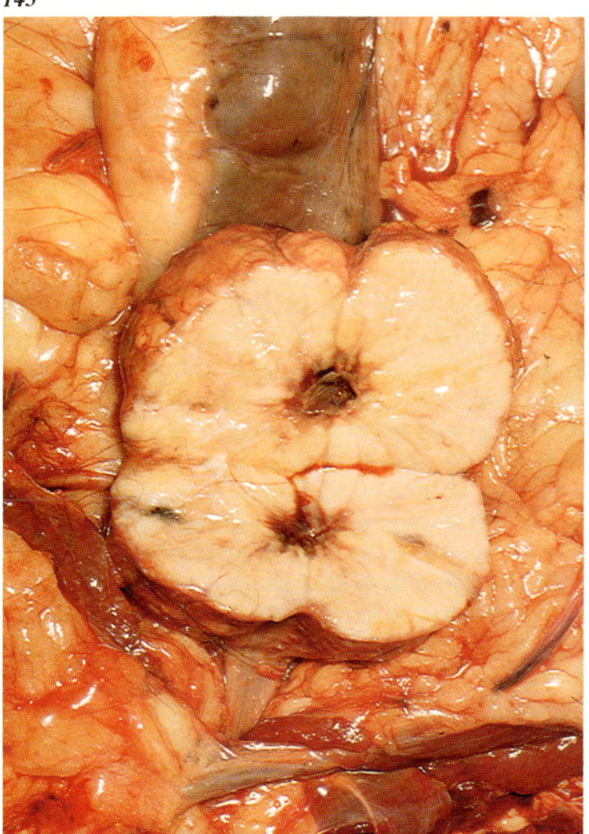

144

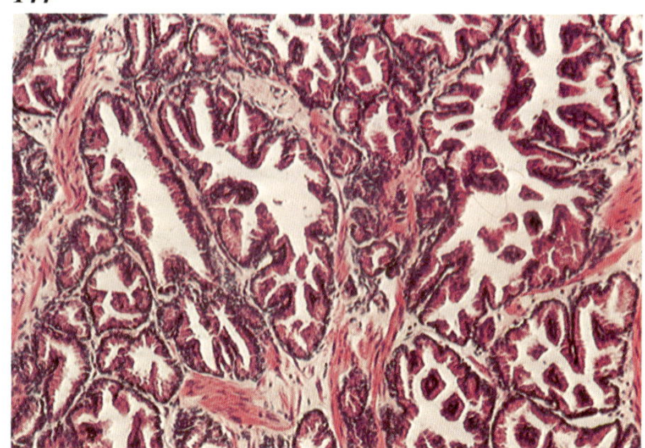

142 *Benign prostatic hyperplasia – dog. The organ has retained its bilobed structure.*

143 *Cut surface of hyperplastic prostate – dog.*

144 *Benign prostatic hyperplasia – dog. H & E.*

Chapter 5
The Urinary System

Lymphosarcomas and tumour metastases are common in the kidney but primary tumours of the urinary system are unusual. Adenomas and embryonal nephromas occur in the kidney, and have been described in all three species, but renal carcinomas are very rare, being found almost exclusively in older dogs. Papillomas and carcinomas arising from the mucosa of the urinary bladder and urethra are seen more frequently than renal tumours in the dog and horse, but are rare in cats.

Renal Adenomas and Carcinomas

Occurrence and gross appearance

These tumours usually arise in the renal cortex in middle-aged or older animals and may become very large before they are diagnosed. Adenomas are well circumscribed, often encapsulated and have a firm, whitish, homogeneous cut surface. Even in large tumours a rim of normal kidney generally remains. Carcinomas are locally invasive and adhesions to surrounding tissues quickly form. Although the tumour starts in one pole of the kidney the entire organ soon becomes replaced by neoplastic tissue (***145***) which is rather dark in colour and has a cut surface mottled by necrosis and haemorrhage. Clinical signs include abdominal enlargement, lethargy, variable appetite and vomiting. The diagnosis can be confirmed by pyelography and exploratory laparotomy.

Histological appearance

Benign tumours are usually papillary cyst adenomas, consisting of large cystic spaces, lined by a branching epithelium. Adenocarcinomas are variable in appearance, consisting either of columnar cells arranged as small, irregular tubules (***146***), or solid sheets containing cystic areas.

Treatment and prognosis

Following nephrectomy the prognosis in animals with renal adenomas should be good. Carcinomas are often impossible to excise completely because of their invasive nature and the prognosis should always be guarded. Local regrowth and metastasis to the liver, lungs and other organs is common, but in some of those cases where metastases were not present at the time of operation, nephrectomy has been successful.

Embryonal Nephromas

Occurrence and gross appearance

These are rare tumours which develop from embryological remnants in the kidney and tend to occur in young animals. They are slowly growing, benign and may become very large before they are diagnosed. They generally replace the entire kidney and appear as irregularly shaped, well encapsulated tumours with a firm, greyish-white cut surface, sometimes containing areas of haemorrhage and necrosis. Diagnosis is the same as for other renal tumours.

Histological appearance

The characteristic feature is the presence of both epithelial and mesenchymal elements, tumours usually consisting of an actively proliferating spindle cell stroma containing irregular acinar structures and glomeruli (*147*). Striated muscle and collagen are commonly found and cartilage and bone can occur.

Treatment and prognosis

If the tumour is very large when diagnosed surgical removal can be difficult but following complete excision the prognosis is favourable.

Transitional Cell Papillomas and Carcinomas

Occurrence and gross appearance

These form the majority of neoplasms of the urinary tract, but are nevertheless rare in cats and horses. Papillomas may be single or multiple and can arise from the mucosa of the bladder or urethra. They are usually less than 1cm in diameter, well circumscribed, fungating, pedunculated nodules which are confined to the mucosa (*148*), the underlying musculature being normal.

Carcinomas are often extensive when first diagnosed and may arise from the bladder (*149*), urethra, renal pelvis (*150*) or ureters, so that in the bladder the wall becomes firm and diffusely thickened, and adhesions form between the serosa and nearby viscera.

Mucosal ulceration with infection and haemorrhage is usual, both papillomas and carcinomas manifesting themselves by dysuria, with pus and blood in the urine, while tumours of the urethra eventually lead to urinary obstruction. Diagnosis may be made by pneumocystography (*151*), endoscopy or exploratory laparotomy.

Histological appearance

Papillomas are well circumscribed, non-invasive and consist of long cones of loose connective tissue covered by a well differentiated transitional epithelium (*153*). Carcinomas are diffusely invasive and show a variety of morphological forms. They consist of a dense fibrous stroma which is heavily infiltrated by small solid rosettes of epithelial cells or definite acinar structures (*152*), or in some cases by keratinising prickle cells, this form being indistinguishable from squamous cell carcinoma.

145 *Renal adenocarcinoma – dog. The entire structure of the affected kidney has been lost.*

146 *Renal adenocarcinoma – dog. H & E.*

147 *Embryonal nephroma – dog. Note the structure resembling glomeruli and tubules. H & E.*

148 *Multiple papillomas of urethra in a dog. There is also evidence of cystitis due to partial urinary retention.*

149 *Transitional cell carcinoma bladder – horse.*

150 *Transitional cell carcinoma of renal pelvis – dog.*

151 *Pneumocystogram showing irregular masses on bladder wall due to transitional cell carcinoma.*

152 *Transitional cell carcinoma of bladder. H & E.*

153 *Papilloma bladder. There is no evidence of infiltration of the underlying connective tissue by the proliferating epithelial cells. H & E.*

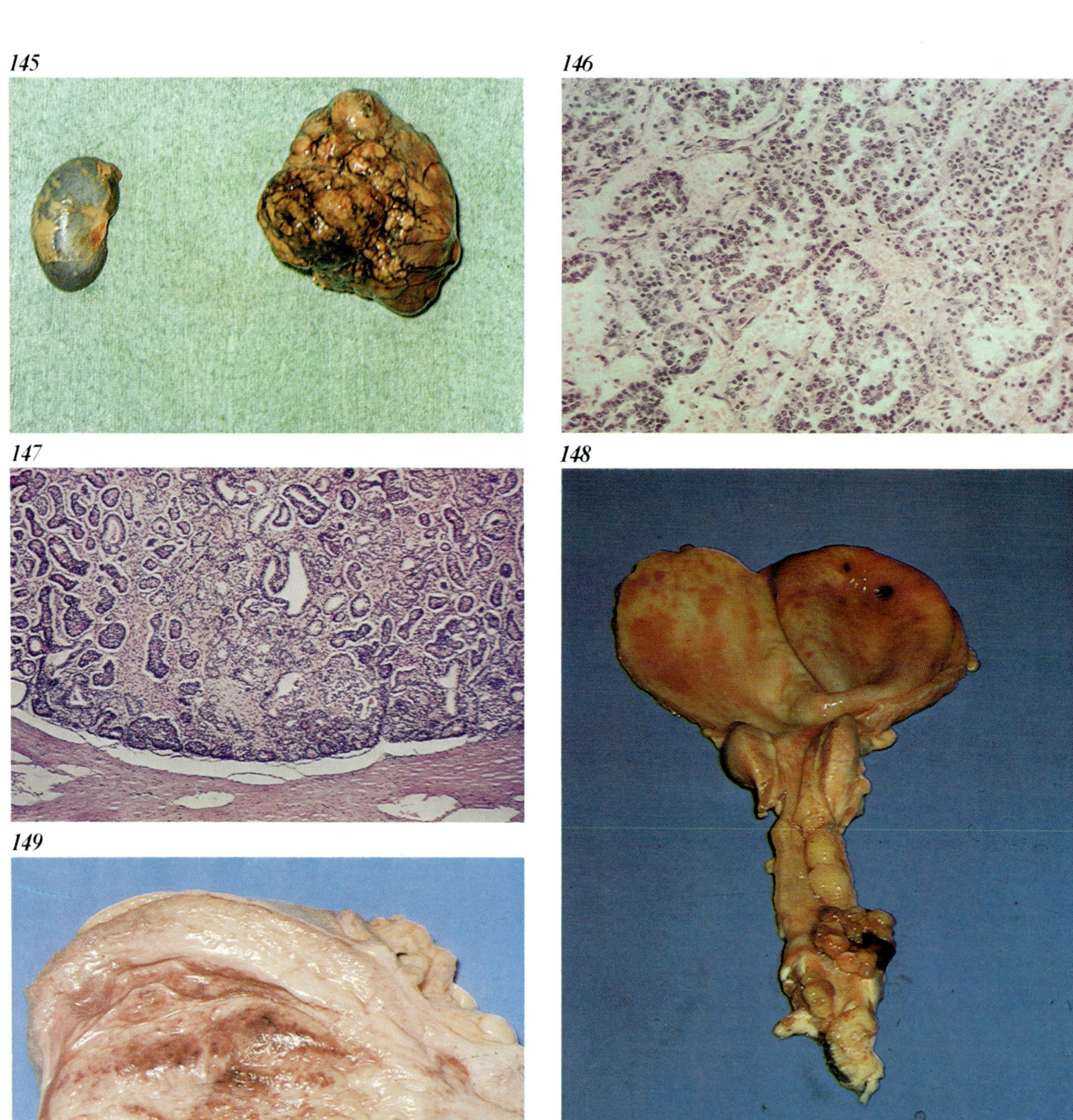

145 **146** **147** **148** **149**

150

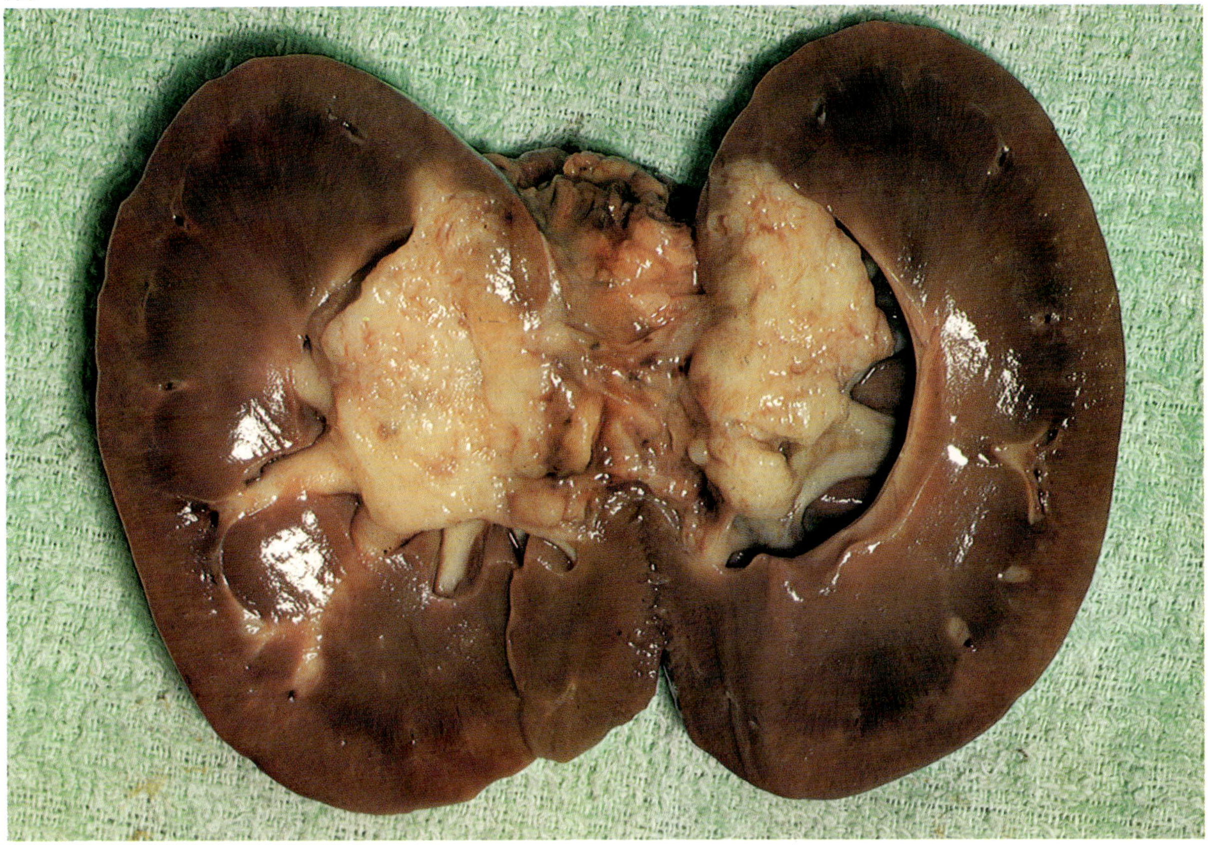

151

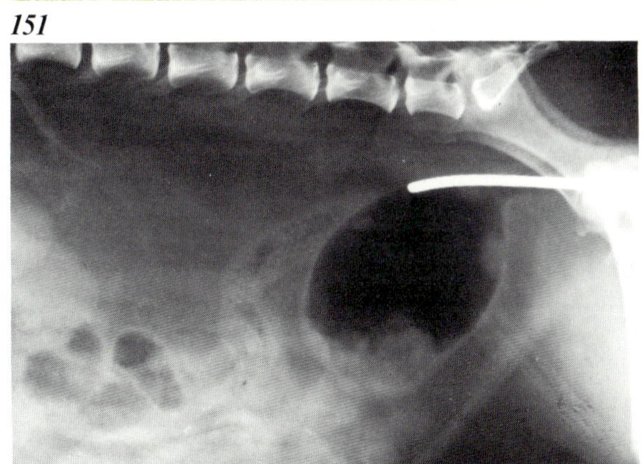

152

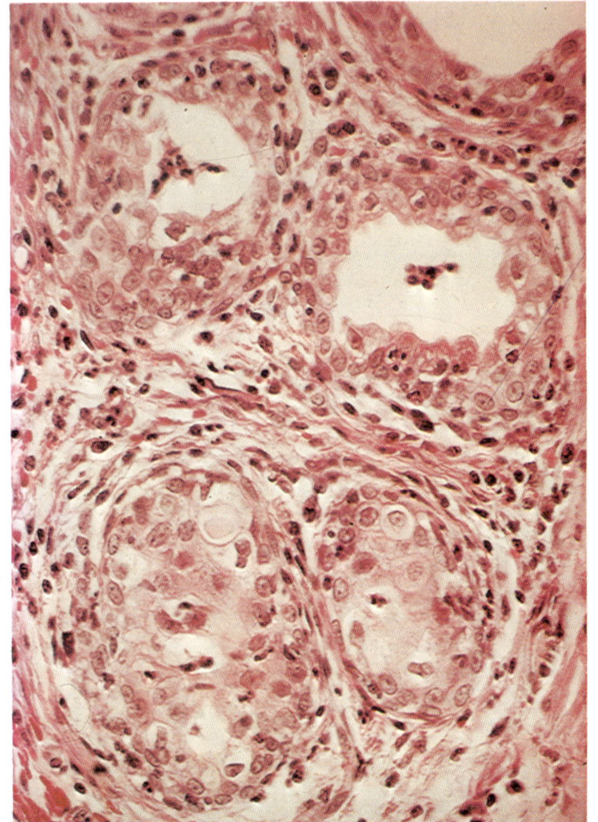

153

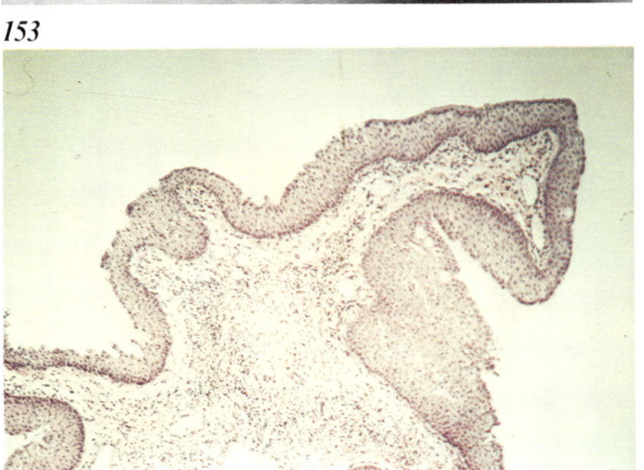

Aetiology
Carcinoma of the bladder can be induced in dogs by the feeding of ß Naphthylamine and certain other chemical carcinogens but the cause of spontaneous tumours is unknown. The development of papillomas may be associated with a chronic, low grade cystitis.

Treatment and prognosis
Surgical excision of solitary papillomas in the bladder is followed by a favourable prognosis although when these are situated in the upper part of the urethra excision is difficult.

The prognosis in animals with carcinomas must always be poor since metastasis, especially to the iliac lymph nodes, is very common. Palliation for up to a few months may be achieved by the intravesicular injection of Thio-tepa at a dose of 2mg/kg B.wt. in 0.3% solution repeated every two weeks for a period of six weeks.

Chapter 6
The Central Nervous System

Tumours of the central nervous system are not rare in animals, although dogs and cats are affected more than horses. In dogs there are breed differences, brachycephalic dogs showing a high incidence of gliomas, especially oligodendrogliomas.

The brain is often the site for secondary neoplasms especially carcinomas (***154***), haemangioendotheliomas, and lymphosarcomas which infiltrate the meninges (***155***). In the dog it has been estimated that metastases account for about one quarter of the total number of tumours in this site.

Clinical signs of space-occupying lesions are extremely variable but may include one or more of the following: dullness, hyperexcitability, tremors and alteration of character, abnormal gait, tilting of the head, circling, difficulty in eating, nystagmus, ptosis, dilated pupils and impaired vision.

TUMOURS OF THE NEURAL ECTODERM

Astrocytomas

These have been recorded in all three species, most cases being seen in old dogs. The most common sites are the cerebrum and the cerebellum. Tumours may be well defined and relatively benign (***156***), or invasive, although metastases have not been recorded.

Microscopically, they consist of well differentiated astrocytes producing parallel bundles or whorls of glial fibres, the number of fibres being variable (***157***). In a few cases 'giant astrocytes' may also be seen while in many cases the tumours contain areas of small, closely packed cells with a very densely staining nucleus and sparse cytoplasm. Tumours in which this type of cell predominates are termed oligodendrogliomas (***158***).

Ependymomas

These tumours are usually well circumscribed and benign (***159***). Histologically they consist of numerous rosettes of columnar cells which are lining cleft-like spaces, the nucleus typically being situated at the pole of the cell nearest to the space (***160***).

Papillomas and Carcinomas of the Choroid Plexus

Papillomas and carcinomas of the choroid plexus occur in the dog and horse, mainly in older animals, the usual site being the lateral or fourth ventricle (***161***). It is difficult to distinguish between benign and malignant types with both being composed of long, branching papillae consisting of a central fibrous core lined by columnar epithelial cells.

154 *Metastatic nodule from a mammary adenocarcinoma in the cerebrum of a dog.*

155 *Lymphosarcomatous infiltration of the cerebellar meninges – cat. H & E.*

156 *Astrocytoma in the fore brain of a dog.*

157 *Astrocytoma – dog. H & E.*

158 *Oligodendroglioma – cat. H & E.*

159 *Ependymoma in the thalamus – dog.*

154

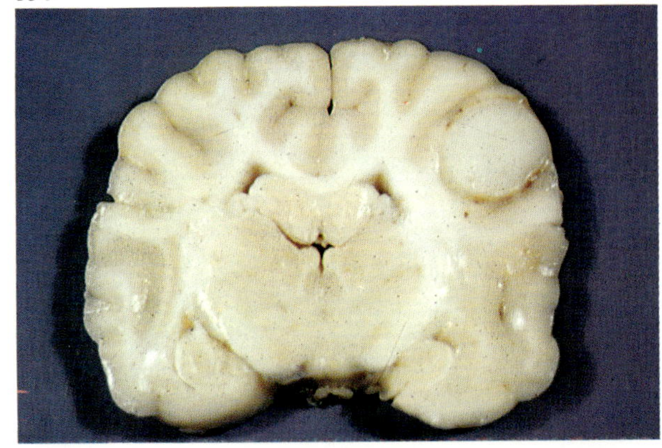

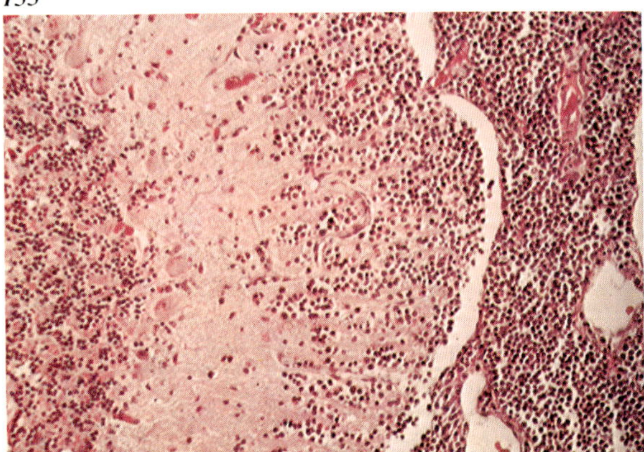

156

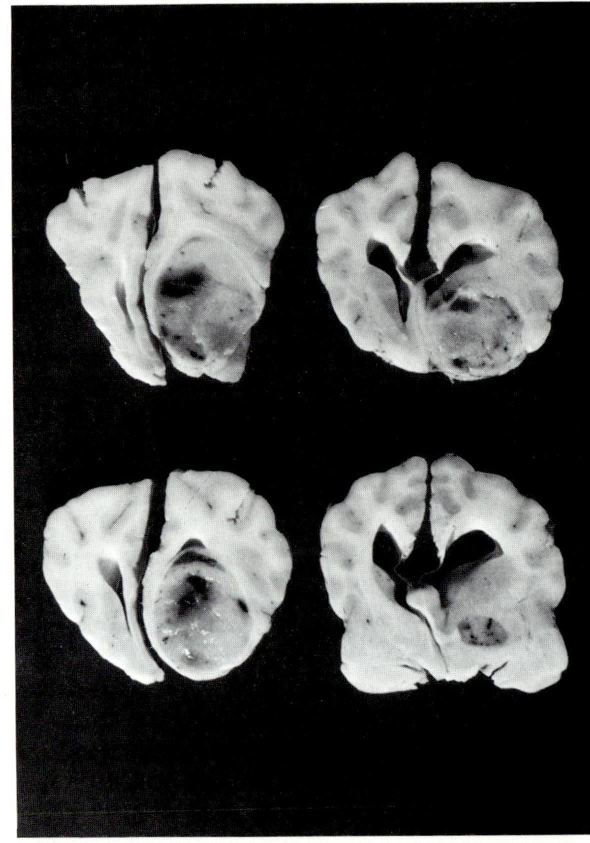

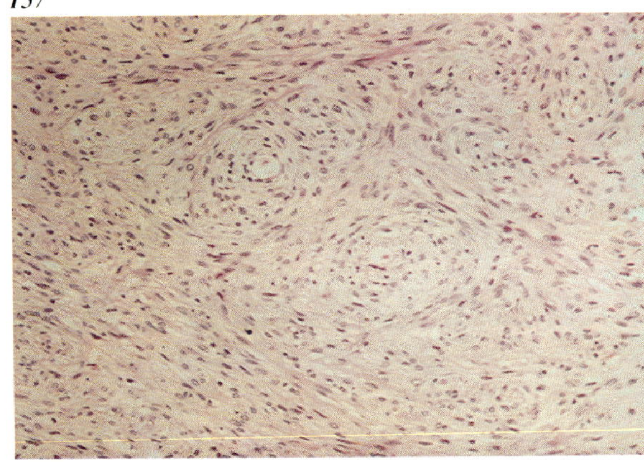

158

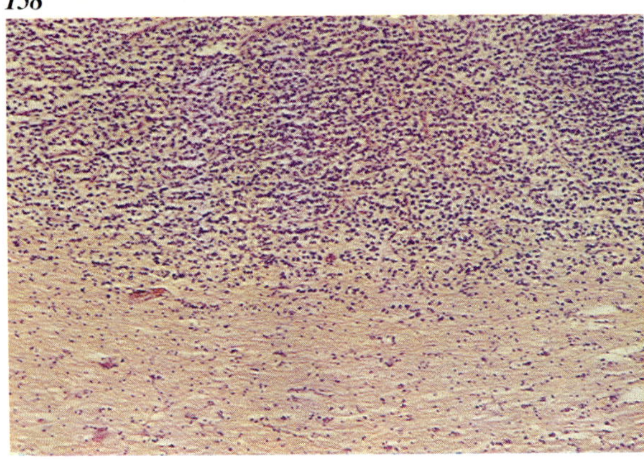

159

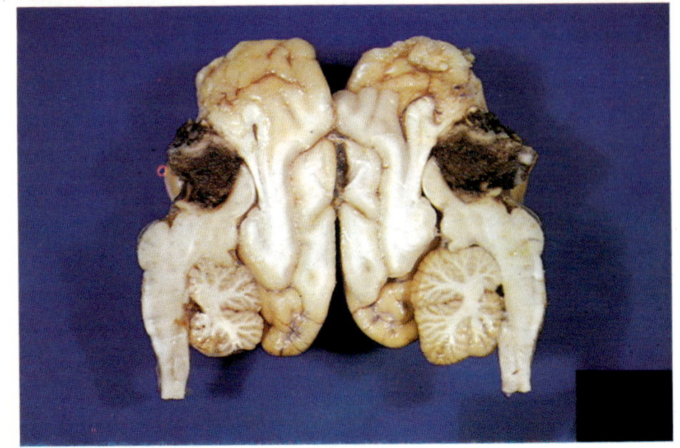

160 *Ependymoma – dog. H & E.*

161 *Plexus papilloma in lateral ventricle – dog.*

160

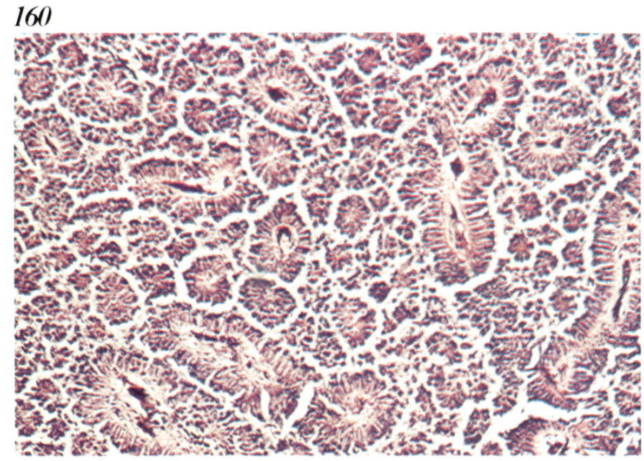

161

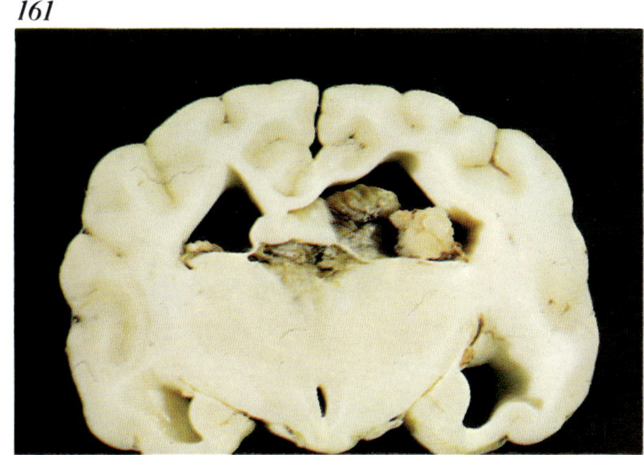

TUMOURS OF THE MESODERM

Meningiomas

Meningiomas have been reported in all three species with a relatively higher incidence in the dog, particularly in old Collies and Alsations. Most arise in the arachnoid mater of the cerebrum or cerebellum and are well circumscribed, encapsulated, firm, white neoplastic masses (***162***). Histologically, spindle-shaped cells are seen forming bundles or tight whorls, some of which may undergo calcification (***163***).

---

162 *Meningioma at base of cerebellum – dog.*

162

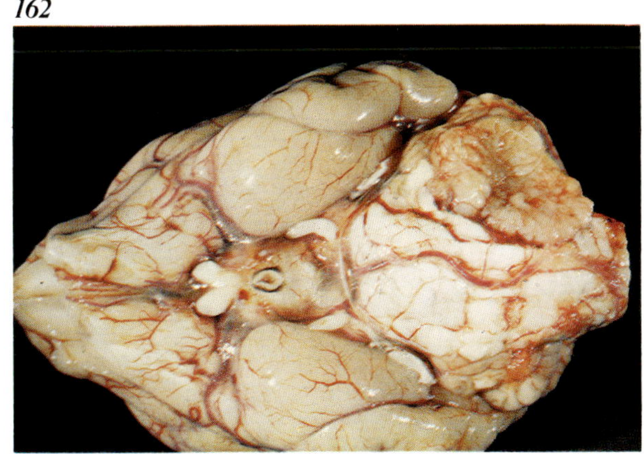

163 *Meningioma – dog. Note the small, spherical zones of calcification. H & E.*

163

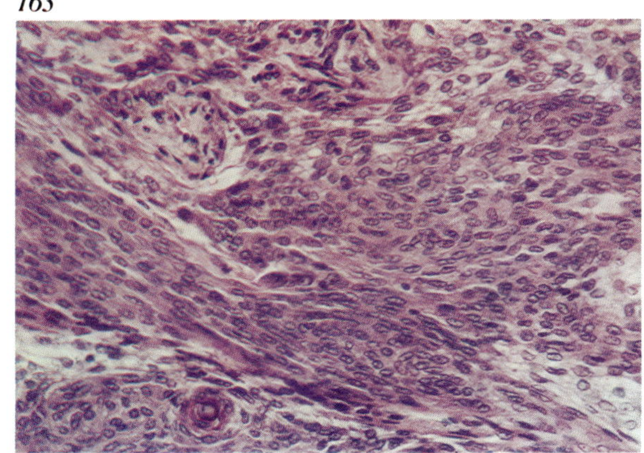

Chapter 7
The Endocrine Glands

Endocrine tumours are characteristically found in old animals. Small benign tumours, often very difficult to distinguish from nodular hyperplasia are commonly seen incidentally on post mortem examination.

Benign tumours may become clinically significant because of pressure necrosis of surrounding tissues or because the neoplastic cells are functional and secrete hormones in an uncontrolled fashion.

Tumours which are of clinical significance occur, in approximate order of incidence, in the adrenal gland, thyroid, pituitary, and aortic body. Oestrogen-producing tumours of the gonads and insulin-producing tumours have been discussed elsewhere, while parathyroid tumours in animals are extremely rare.

Adrenal Cortex Tumours

Occurrence and gross appearance

Small, usually unilateral adenomas measuring up to 2cm in diameter are frequently seen incidentally on post mortem examination of the adrenal cortex of old dogs (***164***), and horses. Larger cortical adenomas, up to several centimetres in diameter, which have completely replaced the adrenal gland also occur, most often in dogs. These tumours are roughly oval, well encapsulated, and are pale brownish yellow in colour. They have a homogeneous, friable cut surface which may contain areas of haemorrhage, while a small remnant of the original adrenal gland is often present at the edge. Most are unilateral, the opposite adrenal being atrophic. Adrenal cortical carcinomas are less common than adenomas and may become very large before they are diagnosed. Again they are unilateral but are non-encapsulated and extremely locally invasive, with infiltration of the neighbouring kidney being common. The tumour is irregular in shape, friable in consistency, and usually contains large areas of liquefactive necrosis. Presenting signs include lethargy, inappetence and abdominal distension, often associated with a large volume of bloody ascitic fluid.

Histological appearance

Both adrenal adenomas and carcinomas are usually derived from the zona fasciculata, and are composed of large, pale staining cells with foamy, vacuolated cytoplasm, arranged as solid lobules surrounded by fibrous tissue septa. The cells have a central, spherical nucleus and cell boundaries are very indistinct (***165***). The degree of malignancy may be difficult to assess although carcinomas tend to consist of smaller, less well differentiated cells, arranged in small solid clumps or as very rudimentary acini covering fine fibrous septa. The cells are hyperchromatic, have sparse cytoplasm, and mitotic figures are common.

Treatment and prognosis

Some adrenal adenomas in dogs are functional and produce cortisol, leading to the development of Canine Cushing's Syndrome (*see page 92*). Surgical removal of the affected gland will lead to complete cure in the majority of these cases.

Animals with adrenal carcinomas must always be given a poor prognosis since surgical removal is extremely difficult due to the diffusely invasive nature of the tumour. Metastases, especially to the liver are common (***166***), and infiltration into the lumen of the vena cava is also a frequent finding.

Phaeochromocytomas

Occurrence and gross appearance

These tumours, which are derived from the cells of the adrenal medulla are rare in all species, but are seen most often in dogs. They are usually unilateral tumours which do not manifest themselves clinically until they are very large (***167***), although a few early cases have been described in which signs of adrenaline release, including bouts of tachycardia and excitability, were noted. More frequently the presenting signs are non-specific and similar to those seen with other large intra-abdominal masses, diagnosis in these cases resting upon exploratory laparotomy.

Grossly these tumours are difficult to distinguish from adrenal carcinomas. They have a soft dark cut surface which may contain extensive areas of haemorrhage.

Histological appearance

Well differentiated tumours have an appearance resembling that of the normal adrenal medulla, the cells being closely packed together in solid lobules and having a central, large, hyperchromatic nucleus and rather sparse cytoplasm (***168***). The adrenal medulla is usually destroyed, but vestiges of it may be seen even in large tumours.

In order to make an exact diagnosis portions of the tumour should be fixed in a dichromate solution, e.g. Zenker's fixative. Following normal histological processing the cells will then contain numerous golden brown granules of chromaffin pigment.

Treatment and prognosis

Since these tumours are frequently very large and may have bled extensively into the abdominal cavity when first detected euthanasia is usually performed following exploratory laparotomy.

164 *Cut surface of adrenal adenoma – dog. Some normal medullary tissue has been preserved.*

165 *Adrenal adenoma – dog. The cells are large and have foamy cytoplasm. H & E.*

166 *Hepatic and pulmonary metastasis from adrenal adenocarcinoma – dog.*

167 *Phaeochromocytoma – dog. This is a large but well circumscribed tumour.*

168 *Phaeochromocytoma – dog. The tumour cells are lining vascular channels yet metastasis is rare. H & E.*

169 *Thyroid adenoma – dog.*

170 *Thyroid adenocarcinoma – dog. The tumour is non-encapsulated, irregular in outline and has metastasised to the lungs.*

171 *Thyroid adenoma. The follicles are well formed and filled with apparently normal colloid – horse. M. S. B.*

172 *Papillary adenocarcinoma of thyroid – dog. H & E.*

173 *Solid thyroid carcinoma – dog. H & E.*

174 *Squamous metaplasia in solid thyroid carcinoma – dog. H & E.*

175 *Mixed thyroid tumour containing bone – dog. H & E.*

164

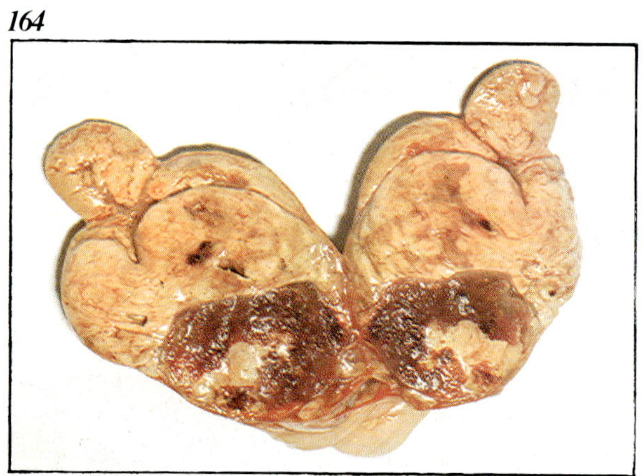

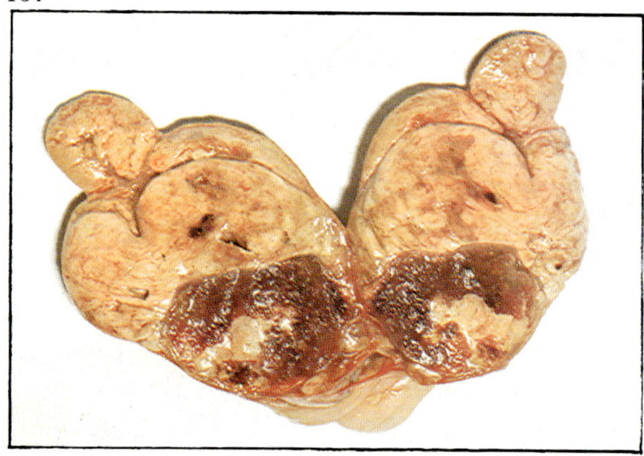

165

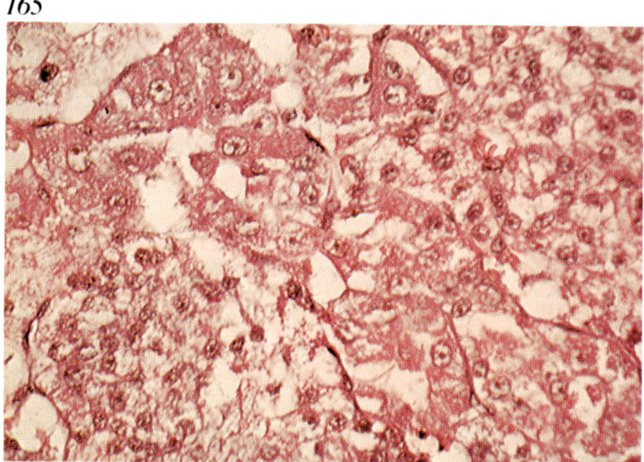

166

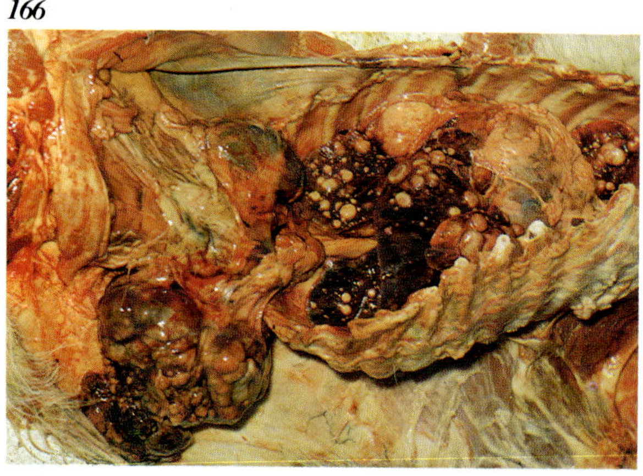

167

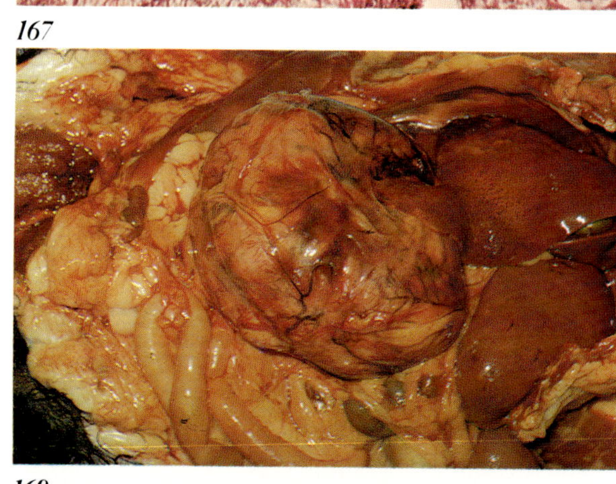

168

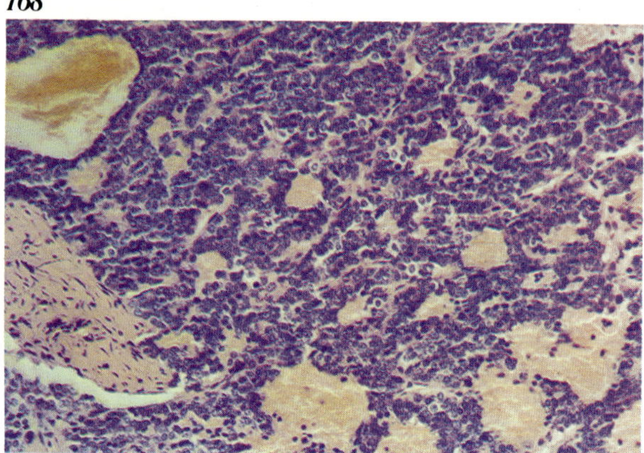

169

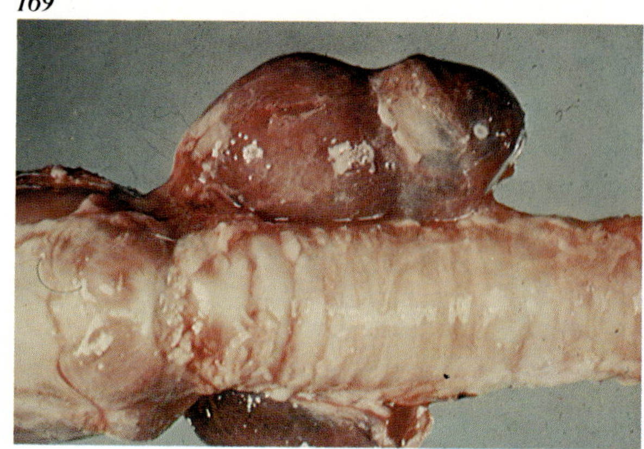

Thyroid Adenomas and Adenocarcinomas

Occurrence and gross appearance

These tumours are seen relatively frequently in the dog and horse, but less commonly in cats. They occur especially in areas where iodine deficiency exists. Thyroid tumours are usually unilateral, although both glands may be involved, and adenomas are found more frequently than carcinomas. Benign tumours are slowly growing and asymptomatic, so that they are usually large when first seen and appear as a firm, roughly oval, well encapsulated and freely mobile mass situated near the middle of the neck, lateral and

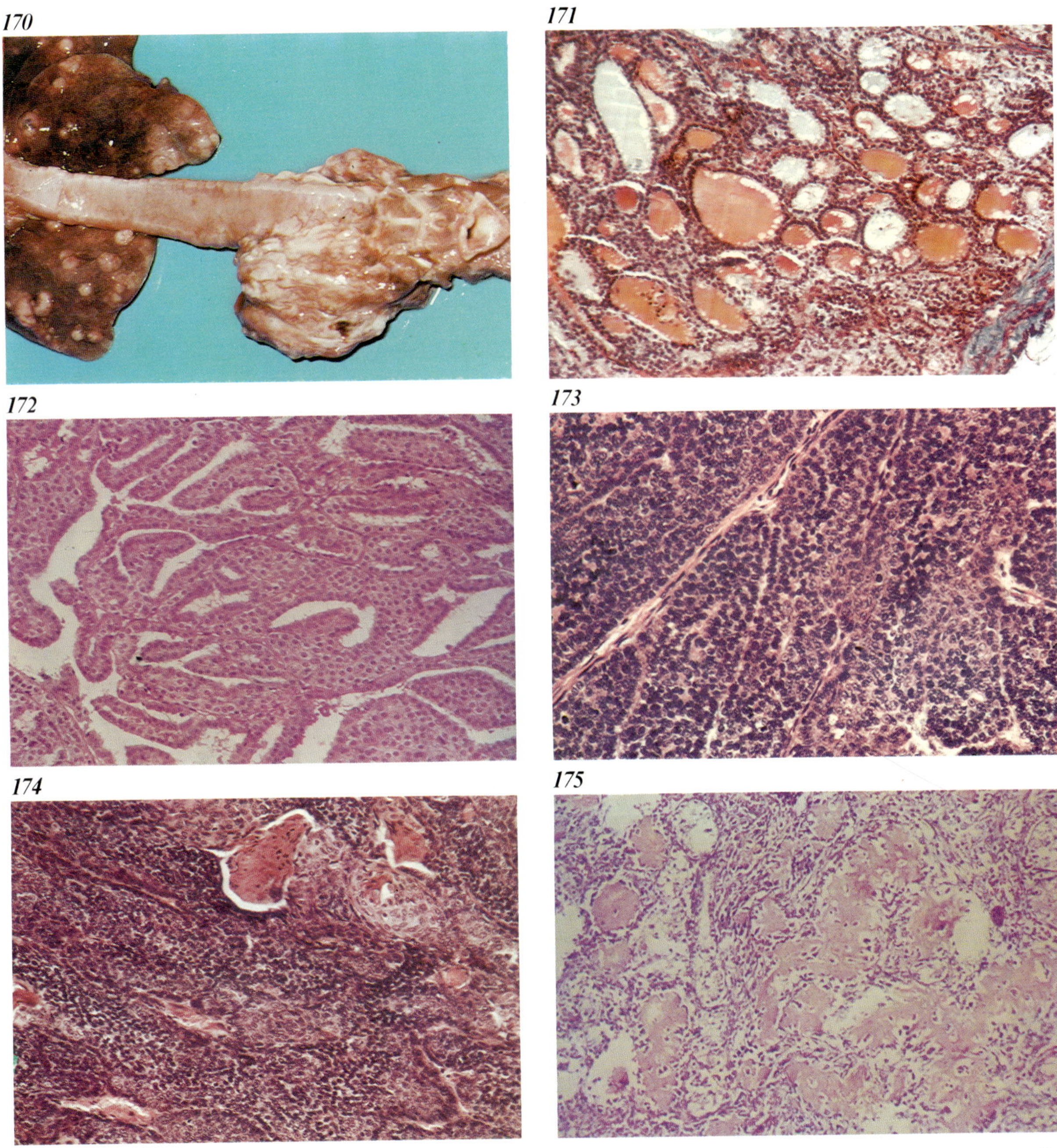

slightly dorsal to the trachea (*169*). They may measure up to 10cm long when presented and have a homogeneous, yellowish-brown cut surface.

Carcinomas grow more rapidly, and are firmly attached to the surrounding tissues. They appear grossly as multinodular, firm, whitish and well vascularised lesions which invade the surrounding musculature and fascia (*170*).

Histological appearance

The histological appearance of benign tumours tends to be rather variable although they are characteristically surrounded by a thick fibrous capsule. Most adenomas consist of well defined follicles, lined by cuboidal epithelial cells and filled with secretion (*171*).

Carcinomas are poorly circumscribed and may show obvious infiltration into the stroma and local vessels. Again the appearance is variable, but commonly the mass is composed of hyperchromatic epithelial cells arranged as branching papillae (*172*) , or rudimentary acini and solid foci (*173*). Areas of colloid may also be present, but are less obvious than in benign tumours. The individual cells in carcinomas tend to be smaller and more hyperchromatic and mitotic figures may be common. Occasionally, squamous metaplasia is apparent in canine thyroid carcinomas (*174*), although care must be taken to distinguish between this and a metastasis from a tonsillar carcinoma. Mixed tumours containing myxomatous tissue, bone or cartilage also occur (*175*).

Aetiology

The observation that thyroid tumours are much commoner in areas of iodine deficiency suggests that abnormal hormone production and follicular hyperplasia may lead to neoplastic transformation. The exact mechanism for this is unknown.

Treatment and prognosis

Benign tumours in dogs and horses can be removed easily, and carry a favourable prognosis. Rarely, tumours may develop in the remaining thyroid gland, when surgical removal leads to a hypoparathyroidism which is difficult to control. In this event the calcium content of the diet should be increased by the administration of calcium lactate.

Carcinomas are usually difficult to remove surgically because of their invasive nature, and thus local recurrence is to be expected. This may however take many months to develop and the prognosis following the removal of histologically malignant tumours is better than the histological appearance would suggest. Local recurrence, and in some cases, pulmonary metastasis may eventually occur however. This process can possibly be retarded, although not prevented, by the daily administration of 60–180mg thyroid by mouth.

Pituitary Adenomas

Occurrence and gross appearance

Benign pituitary tumours are much commoner than malignant and are found most often in the dog, although they are also seen in horses. The condition is very rare in cats.

In the dog most tumours develop in the pars distalis of the pituitary and some of them may be functional, secreting especially ACTH. In these cases, the tumour is manifested by the development of 'Canine Cushing's Syndrome', clinical signs including polydipsia, abdominal distension, lethargy, and a progressive bilateral alopecia which spreads up the flanks from the ventral abdomen and hind limbs (*176*).

The adrenal glands are bilaterally enlarged due to hyperplasia of the zona fasciculata at the expense of the remainder of the gland (*177*). In the horse tumours develop mainly in the intermediate part of the pituitary. In this species and in dogs with non-functional tumours the clinical signs consist of lethargy, rough dry coat and partial or complete blindness. Atrophy of the gonads and adrenals occurs and destruction of the neurohypophysis can lead to diabetes insipidus.

Pituitary tumours all tend to have a similar gross appearance, consisting of a firm, roughly spherical, smooth mass, usually measuring 0.5–3cm in diameter (*178*), but sometimes being larger, situated just behind the optic chiasma. Most tumours are benign, and are clearly defined from the surrounding brain tissue, although they are not encapsulated.

Histological appearance

In the dog, adenomas of the chromophobe cells are the most common, acidophil and basophil tumours being unusual. They are composed of large epithelial cells, closely packed together and arranged as solid sheets (*179*), lining thin connective tissue septa where they may produce acinar structures, or forming rosettes around blood vessels (*180*). The cells have a central, open nucleus containing a number of small chromatin granules, abundant granular cytoplasm and indistinct cell boundaries. Special staining techniques (e.g. Barrett's) may enable the different types of tumour to be distinguished. Figure ***181*** shows the appearance of a chromophobe adenoma, the cells being pale greyish-blue in colour. Using this method acidophils stain bright red and basophils blue.

Treatment and prognosis

These tumours are characteristically slowly growing and do not metastasise, but because of their anatomical site the prognosis is always poor once clinical signs develop.

176 *Alopecia of the flanks and abdominal distension in a Boxer with Canine Cushing's Syndrome.*

177 *Hyperplasia of zona fasciculata of adrenals in 'Canine Cushing's Syndrome'. The zona glomerulosa has been obliterated. H & E.*

178 *Pituitary adenoma – dog. This tumour can be seen impinging upon the optic chiasma.*

179 *Pituitary adenoma – solid sheets of cells – dog. H & E.*

180 *Pituitary adenoma – rosettes around blood vessels – dog. H & E.*

181 *Chromophobe adenoma of pituitary gland – dog. Barrett's stain.*

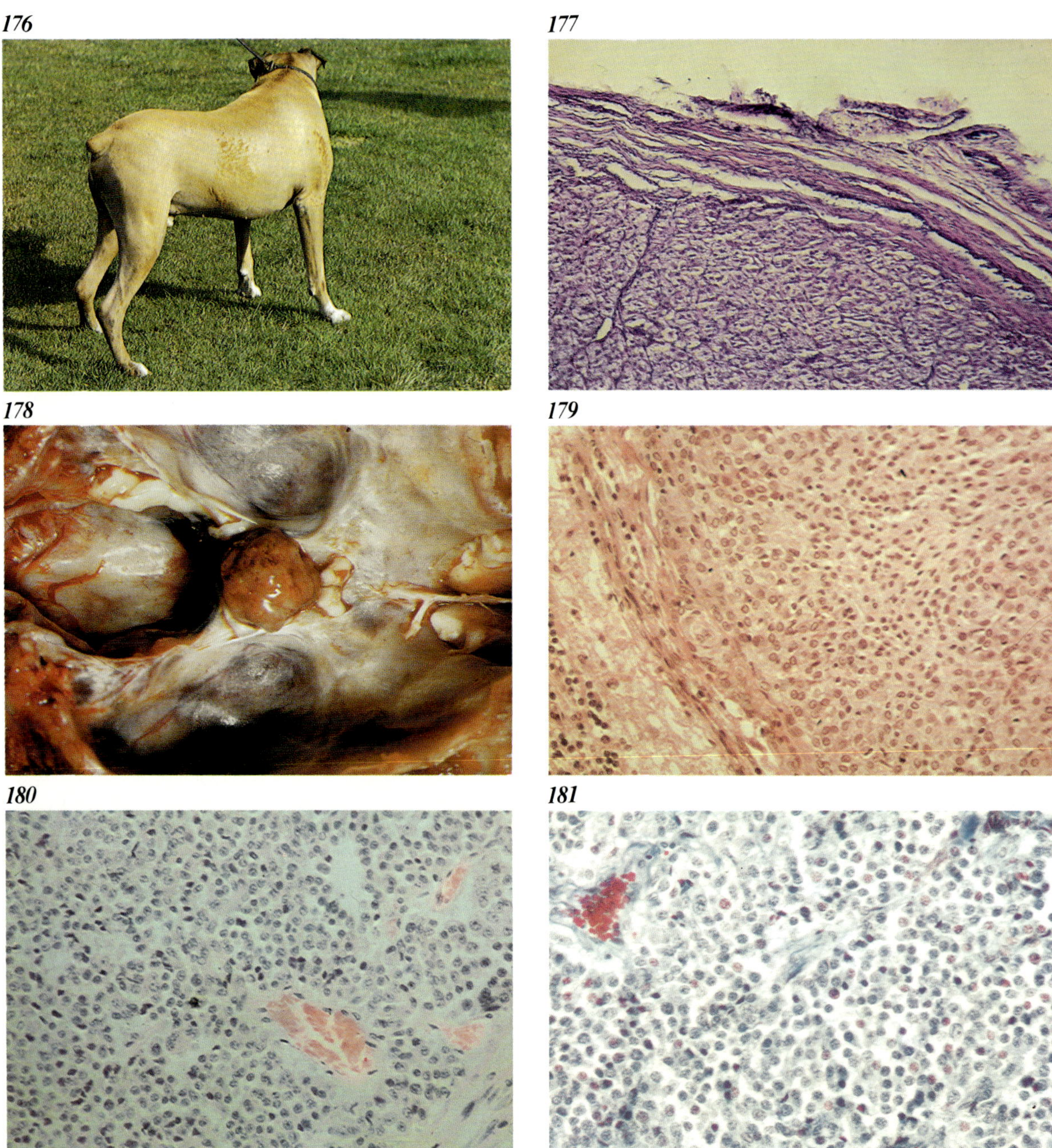

Aortic Body (Heart Base) Tumours

Occurrence and gross appearance

This tumour is found exclusively in old dogs, especially Boxers, the usual site being at the base of the heart between the aorta and the pulmonary artery. Signs of cardiac insufficiency, including pulmonary oedema and congestion of the liver, are often present and the radiographic appearance is of a mass associated with the heart, usually in the dorsal aspect but sometimes in the anterior mediastinum. The gross appearance is of an encapsulated, reddish-brown or pale yellow, lobulated mass with a firm or rubbery consistency (***182***).

Histological appearance

The tumour is composed of a fibrous stroma enclosing tumour cells which are round or polyhedral and which are lining cleft-like spaces (***183***). Mononucleate giant cells can occur and invasion of blood vessels and the capsule is frequent.

It should be noted that some tumours which occur in this site are derived from ectopic thyroid tissue and have a similar histological appearance to other thyroid tumours (*see page 91*).

Treatment and prognosis

Treatment has not been attempted due to the inaccessible nature of the mass. Metastasis, especially to the lungs and myocardium is common and the prognosis is consequently very poor.

Carotid Body Tumours

These tumours occur at the bifurcation of the carotid artery and their gross and histological appearance resembles that of aortic body tumours.

182 *Aortic body (heart base) tumour in a seven-year-old Boxer dog.*

183 *Aortic body (heart base) tumour. H & E.*

183

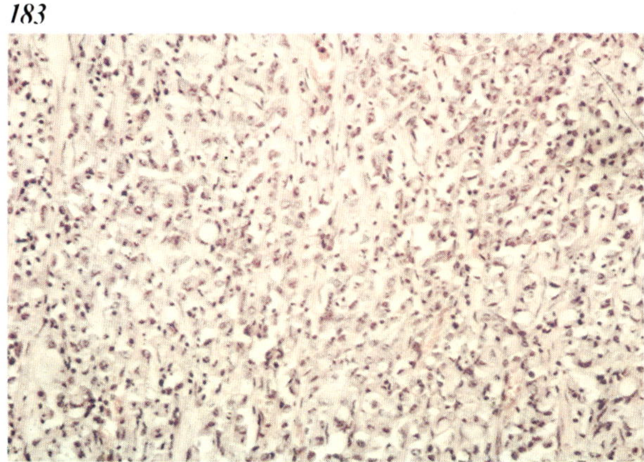

182

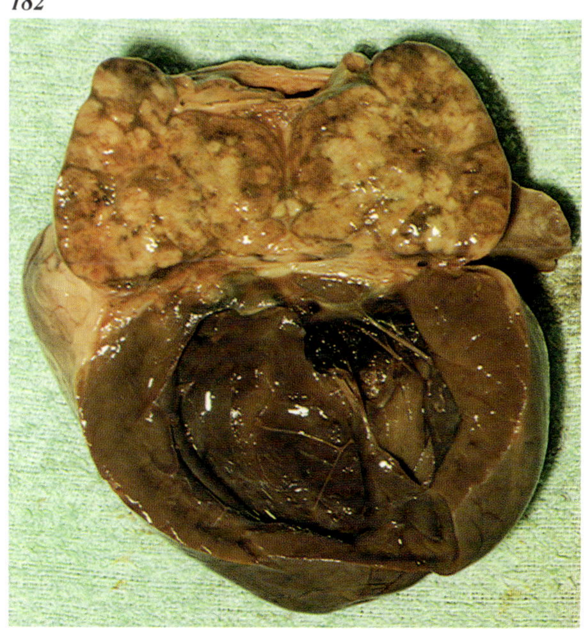

Chapter 8
The Bones and Joints

Osteosarcomas

Occurrence and gross appearance

Osteosarcomas are seen most often in the dog, infrequently in the cat, where they are found mainly in old animals, and rarely in horses. In the dog and cat the tumour usually occurs in the metaphysis of a long bone (***184***), sometimes in the ribs, and in the bones of the skull (***185***). It is much more common in the giant breeds of dog (*e.g. Great Dane*) than in dogs weighing less than 15kg. In the horse, osteosarcomas have been described only in the bones of the head.

Osteosarcomas usually manifest themselves by lameness, followed by swelling of the affected bone. Particularly common sites for development are the proximal humerus, the distal radius and the proximal tibia. Metastasis to the lungs occurs sooner or later in more than 90% of animals with tumours of the limb bones, but metastasis to local lymph nodes only occurs in about 10% of cases. Metastasis from tumours of the head bones is unusual.

On radiography tumours may be mainly osteolytic (***186***) or osteosclerotic (***187***). Frequently there is cortical destruction and formation of periosteal new bone to give a 'sunburst' appearance. The differential diagnosis, which is often difficult on radiographical evidence alone, is from other bone tumours or osteomyelitis due to tuberculosis, blastomycosis, coccidioidomycosis, actinomycosis or other bacterial infection (***188***). Radiographical evidence of lung metastasis is not common when the animal is first presented.

Gross examination of the affected bone reveals severe distortion of its normal shape, with thinning or even complete destruction of the cortex. Often the bone is easy to cut and the marrow cavity is filled with a rather friable, whitish or pink homogeneous tissue, containing a variable amount of cancellous bone. Similar tissue is seen penetrating through the cortex and forming large tumour masses in the surrounding soft tissues (***189***). Cysts and haemorrhages are frequent and areas of necrosis may be found in the larger tumours.

Histological appearance

By definition, an osteosarcoma is a tumour which forms neoplastic osteoid or new bone or both, the osteoid being produced directly by the malignant osteoblasts (***190***). The amount of osteoid in any given tumour can vary considerably however, and most limb tumours tend to be rather poorly differentiated, consisting of sheets of hyperchromatic, polygonal cells which in some areas are closely applied to irregular foci of osteoid.

184 *Osteosarcoma, distal radius and ulna. This is the most common single site.*

185 *Osteosarcoma of maxilla causing compression of the globe.*

186 *Rapidly growing osteolytic osteosarcoma – the radiograph on the right was taken three weeks after that on the left.*

184

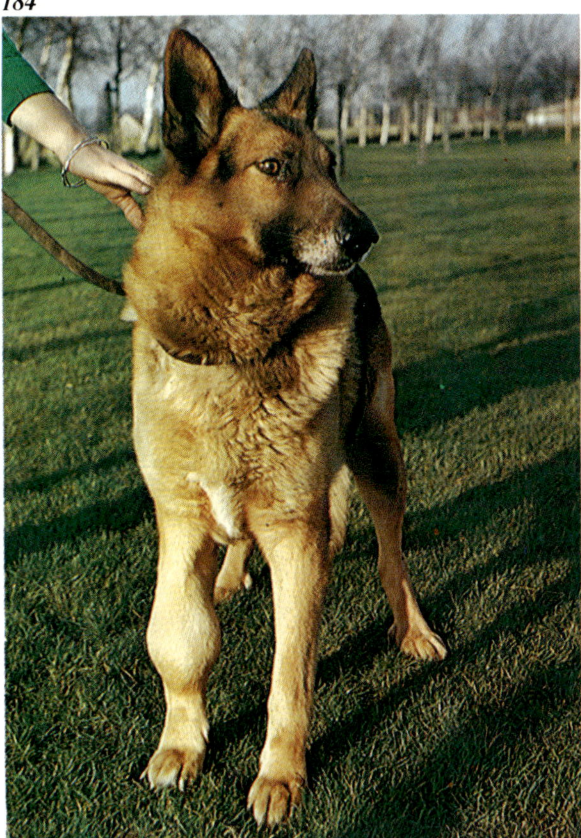

185

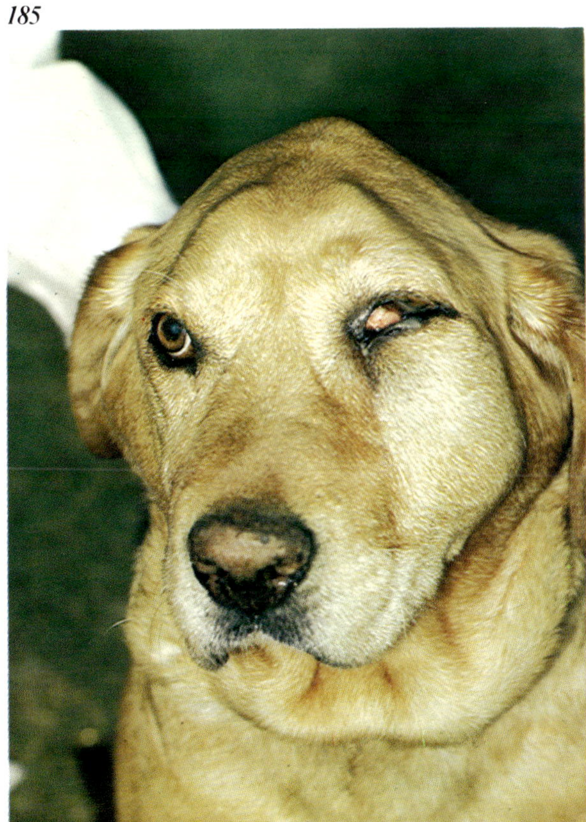

186

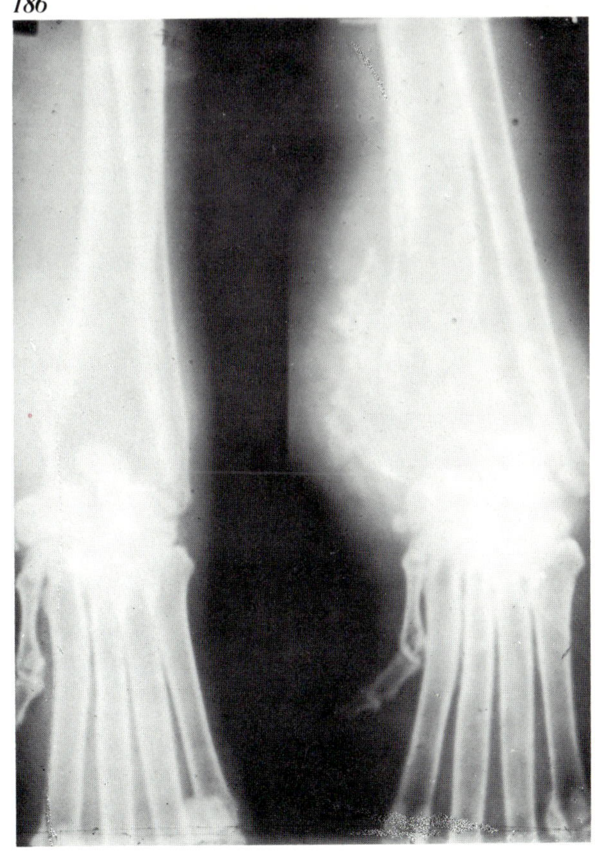

187

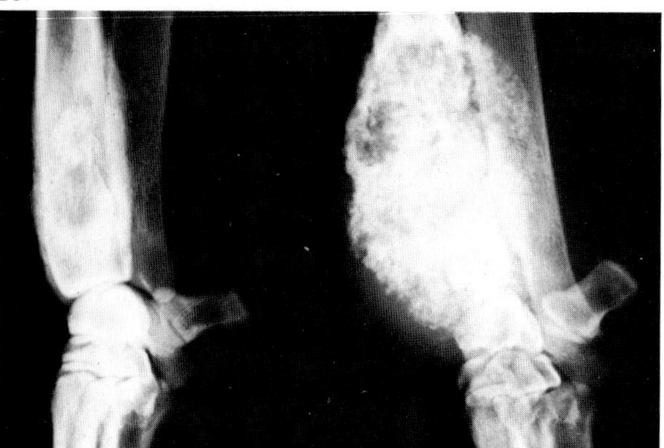

188

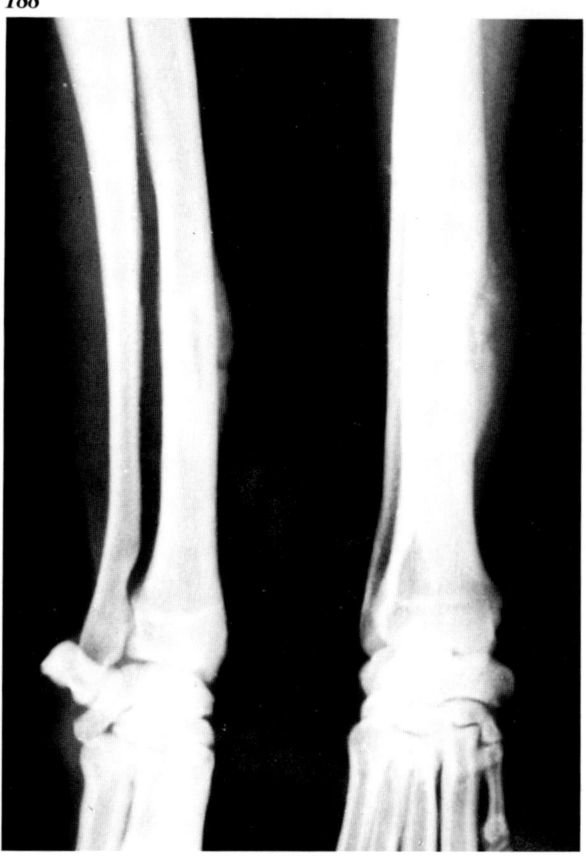

187 *Slowly growing osteosclerotic osteosarcoma – the radiograph on the right was taken five months after that on the left.*

188 *Osteomyelitis at junction of middle and posterior thirds of radius. The distinguishing feature in this case is the presence of an obvious sequestrum – Labrador Retriever.*

Tumours consisting largely of fibroblasts or chondroblasts, with relatively little true osteoid are seen on occasion (***191***). In general, tumours arising in the membrane bones of the head in dogs are much better differentiated than those in the limbs or ribs. Periosteal, non-neoplastic new bone formation is seen as a result of lifting of the periosteum by the neoplastic tissue in most tumours.

Aetiology

Unknown. The possibility exists that in some strains of Great Dane and Wolfhounds there may be a genetic predisposition to the tumour.

Treatment and prognosis

The prognosis is poor. Treatment of the primary tumour by X-irradiation up to 5,000R from a linear accelerator quickly abolishes pain and reduces the rate of growth of the tumour (***192***), but the effect is only palliative. Surgical excision from bones of the cranium is usually followed by local recurrence within a few months and most dogs which have a limb amputed develop lung metastases within six months (***193***).

Benign Tumours of Bone

Benign osteoblastoma has been described in a cat and so-called 'osteomas' occur, particularly on the head of dogs and horses. Some of those which recur after surgical removal can be controlled for long periods of time by fractionated X-irradiation to a total dose of 4,000R.

Chondromas and Chondrosarcomas

Occurrence and gross appearance

These tumours are rare in all three species, but are seen most often in the dog, where they tend to develop more frequently in the membrane bones. True chondromas are very rare, but many chondrosarcomas are of only low grade malignancy.

Chondrosarcomas appear as firm, non-painful masses on the pelvis, bones of the face, ribs (***194***), vertebrae, scapula and some other sites. On section masses of bluish-white cartilage are seen, sometimes containing areas of cavitation, whilst radiographic examination reveals the presence of irregular, mottled and calcified areas, often with a blurred appearance (***195***). Erosion of the cortex is usual, although there is little periosteal reaction.

Histological appearance

All degrees of differentiation occur, the more benign tumours having an abundant cartilaginous matrix (***196***) whilst malignant tumours contain closely packed cells with plump, frequently multiple, nuclei. Mitotic figures are common in the more malignant tumours.

Treatment and prognosis

The prognosis depends on the degree of malignancy. Low grade chondrosarcomas may grow very slowly for a period of several years, and show no tendency towards metastasis, whilst the more malignant tumours grow rapidly and metastasise readily to the lungs. Attempts at local excision of even low grade chondrosarcomas usually result in local recurrence but amputation can result in cures.

Fibrosarcomas

Occurrence and gross appearance

Fibrosarcoma is a primary malignant tumour of bone which arises from the endosteum, and in which there is no osteoid or new bone formation. The tumour is uncommon in the dog and cat, and rare in horses. Lameness, with pain and swelling over the metaphysis of a long bone, are the usual presenting signs and the gross appearance frequently resembles osteosarcoma. The radiographical appearance of early cases shows osteolysis with minimal periosteal reaction (***197***). More advanced cases may show large osteolytic lesions or a 'moth-eaten' appearance of the cortex.

Histological appearance

As for fibrosarcomas elsewhere. Foci of non-neoplastic new bone may be found in some fields.

Treatment and prognosis

Since fibrosarcomas do not metastasise so readily, the prognosis following amputation is more favourable than that for osteosarcoma.

189 *Cut surface of osteosarcoma of distal radius – dog. Spicules of new bone being produced at right angles to the shaft give the typical 'sunburst' appearance.*

190 *Well differentiated osteosarcoma with an abundant osteoid matrix. Picro polychrome stain.*

191 *Osteosarcoma containing large areas of cartilage. Alcian blue stain.*

192 *Loss of hair and skin pigmentation following 5,000R X-irradiation to an osteosarcoma of the distal radius in a Great Dane.*

193 *'Cannon ball' metastasis in lungs from osteosarcoma of radius.*

189

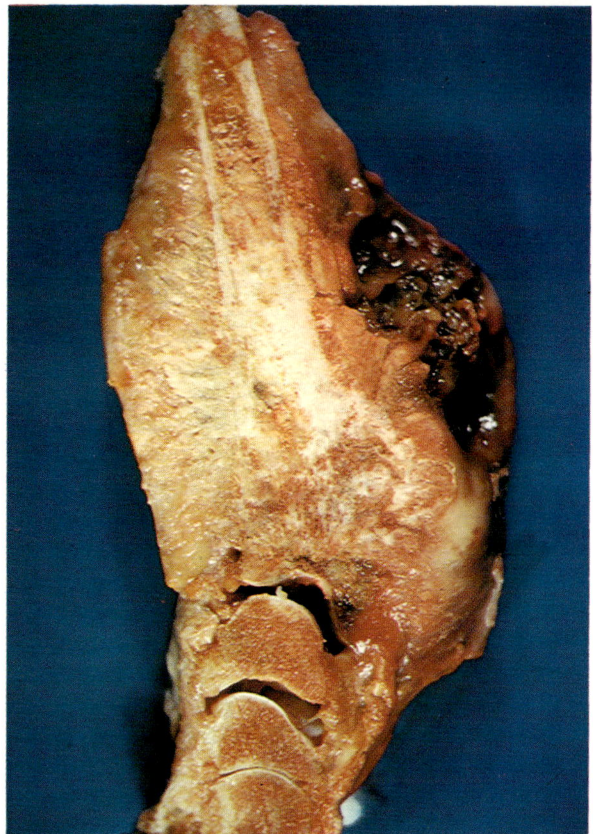

190

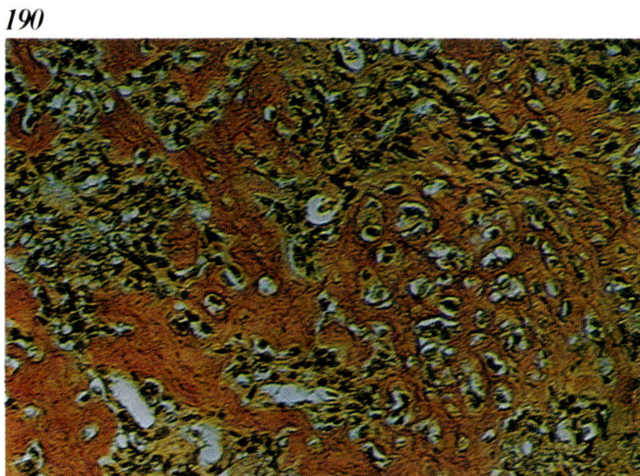

191

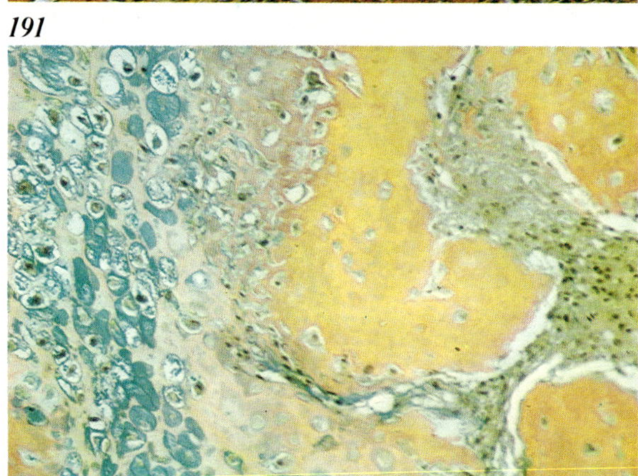

192

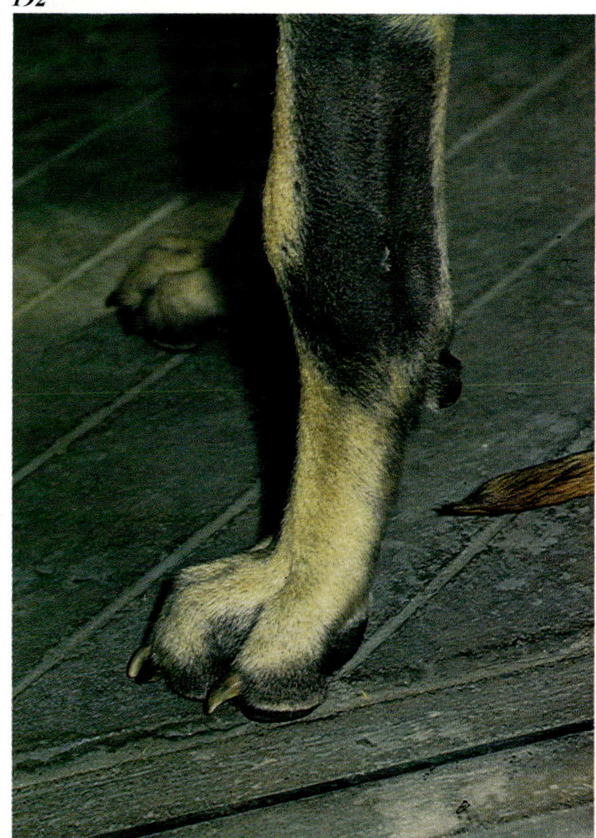

193

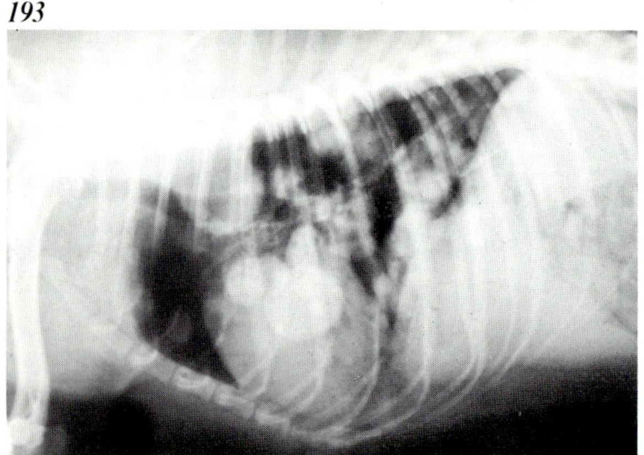

194

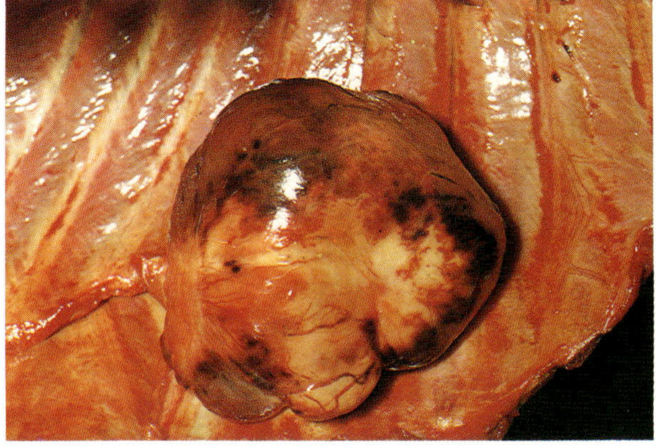

195

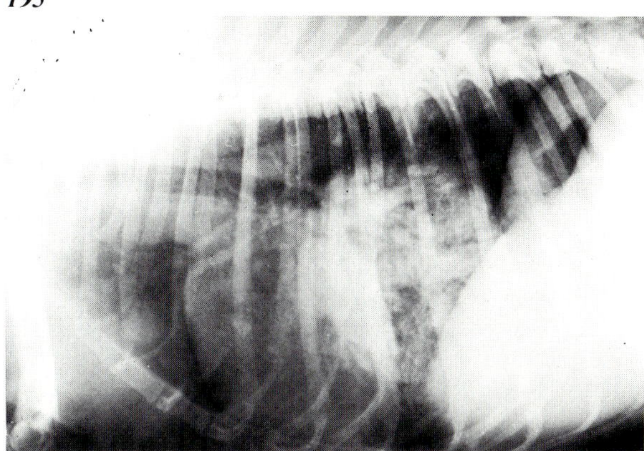

196

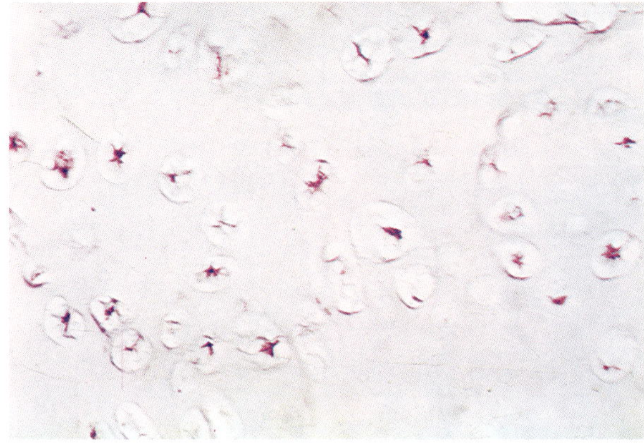

197

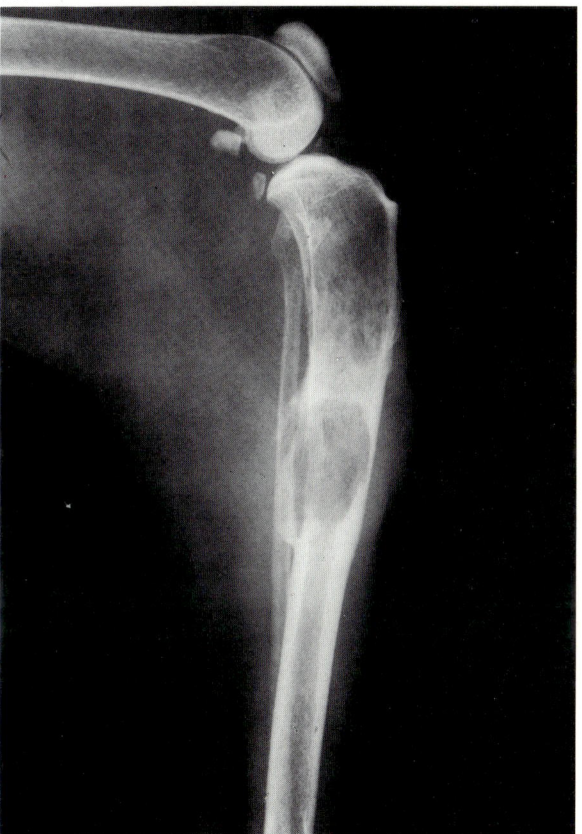

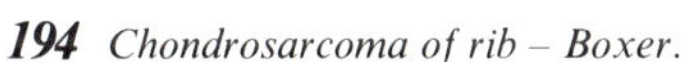

194 *Chondrosarcoma of rib – Boxer.*

195 *Radiographic appearance of chondrosarcoma of the rib – dog.*

196 *Chondroma from the rib of a 10-year-old Yorkshire terrier. H & E.*

197 *Radiograph of fibrosarcoma in the proximal third of the tibia in a 12-year-old cat. Note the clearly defined edge of the lesion and the relative absence of new bone.*

UNCOMMON TUMOURS OF BONE

Malignant Haemangioendothelioma

As seen in the dog the tumour is very destructive and metastasises widely. The histological features are similar to those seen in other parts of the body.

Plasma Cell Myeloma

This tumour, occurring in the dog and horse, originates in the bone marrow where it produces a 'punched out' appearance in the affected bone on radiographic examination. Diagnosis can be made by examination of aspirates of bone marrow stained by methyl green pyronin. The presence of more than 10% plasma cells indicates a positive diagnosis of myeloma. In some tumours 100% of plasma cells are present.

Hypergammaglobulinaemia is found in some cases, leading to the presence of abnormal protein in the urine and renal amyloidosis.

Tumours Metastatic to the Skeleton

It is likely that many metastatic tumours in the skeleton remain undiagnosed. The main records in the dog relate to metastases from tumours of mammary gland, lung and thyroid, the humerus frequently being involved. Both osteolytic and osteosclerotic changes are seen on radiography, sometimes with periosteal new bone formation (***198***).

198

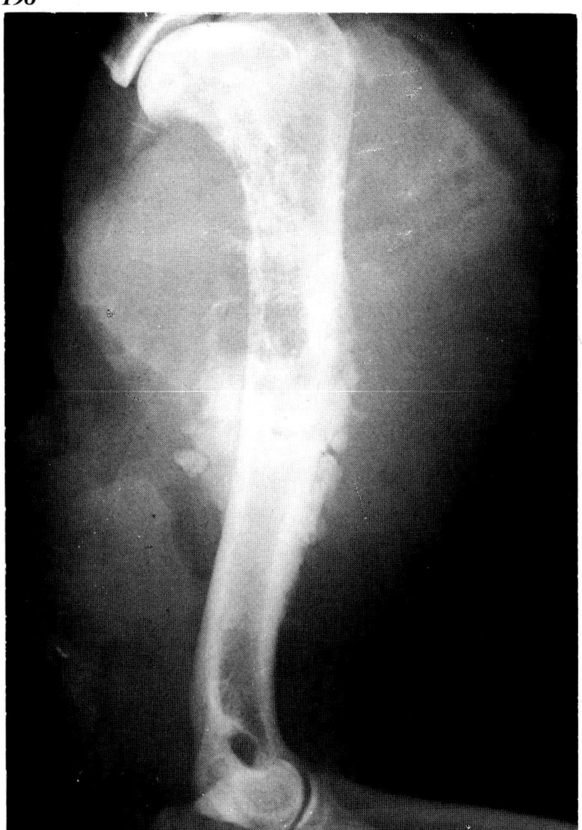

198 *Radiograph of secondary mammary carcinoma in the upper humerus of a seven-year-old Collie.*

Synoviomas and Synoviosarcomas

Benign synoviomas in animals are extremely rare, with most cases having arisen in tendon sheaths. Histological examination shows numerous clefts and cyst-like spaces lined by plump, oval, mesothelial cells.

Synoviosarcomas, arising from joint capsules or tendon sheaths, are also rare, but have been described in dogs and cats, where they generally arise in the region of the stifle or hock.

Diagnosis requires samples from various parts of the tumour, with spindle cells, plump epithelioid cells, and multinucleate giant cells being seen (***199***). Well differentiated tumours may also contain pseudoglandular areas with distinct spaces or clefts (***200***).

Rhabdomyomas and Rhabdomyosarcomas

These are extremely rare tumours which have been described arising from the muscle masses of the limbs and myocardium. They are derived from striated muscle and consist of long, thick multinucleate cells within which cross striations can be demonstrated by the phosphotungstic acid haematoxylin stain.

NON-NEOPLASTIC TUMOUR-LIKE LESIONS

Bone Cysts

Solitary bone cysts are rare, most cases having been described in young dogs. Radiography shows an egg-shell thin bone with ridging on the medullary surface (***201***). Treatment is by curettage, with internal or external fixation to prevent fracture. Packing with bone chips has also been advocated.

Multiple Cartilaginous Exostoses

'Multiple cartilaginous exostoses' is a rare disease involving bones of cartilaginous origin and has been described in all three species. It is manifested by the development of numerous exostoses composed of a large central mass of spongy bone covered by hyaline cartilage (***202** and **203***).

199 *Synoviosarcoma from the hock region of a cat. Note the large number of multinucleate giant cells. H & E.*

200 *Synoviosarcoma from the stifle of a cat. The main feature is the cleft-like spaces lined by flattened cells. H & E.*

201 *Solitary bone cyst in the distal radius of a young Wolfhound. Angiography shows no malignant features.*

202 *Radiographic appearance of multiple cartilaginous exostoses on the vertebrae and ribs – Shetland Collie.*

203 *Cut surface of multiple cartilaginous exostoses. Each nodule consists of a central mass of cancellous bone covered by a thin rim of cartilage.*

204 *Large melanoma of gum in a nine-year-old black and brown mongrel dog.*

205 *Cut surface of oral melanoma – dog.*

206 *Largely amelanotic melanoma involving most of the hard palate in a Scottish Terrier.*

207 *Canine oral melanoma. H & E.*

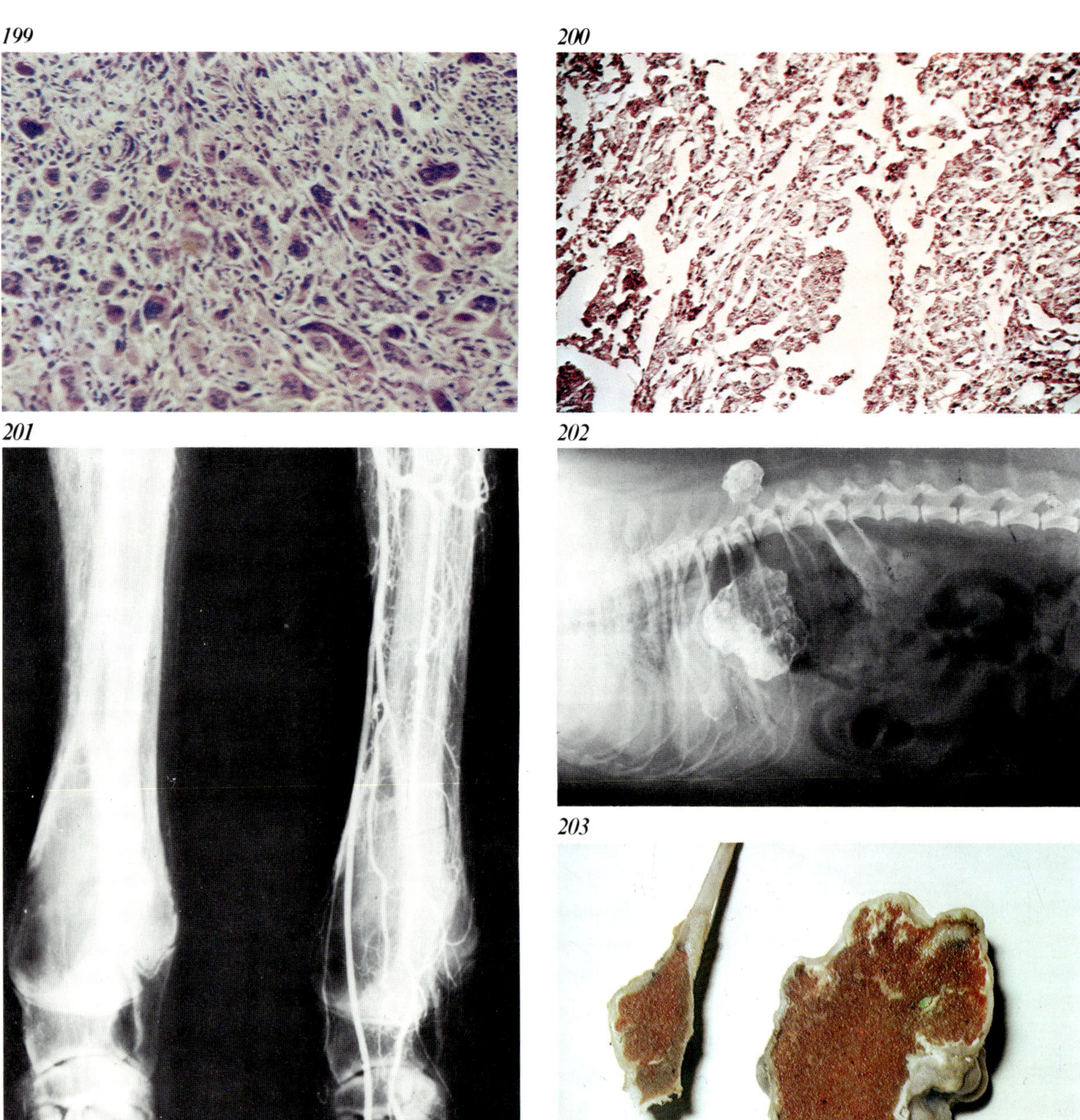

Chapter 9
The Alimentary Tract

Most tumours of the alimentary tract are found in the buccal cavity of the dog and cat, neoplasms in this site being rare in horses. In the dog malignant melanomas are the commonest single tumour type, with squamous cell carcinomas, fibrosarcomas and reticulum cell sarcomas being seen less frequently. In cats the great majority of tumours in the mouth are squamous cell carcinomas, although fibrosarcomas are also found on occasion. Benign tumours are unusual in the mouth but multiple viral papillomas with a gross and histological appearance similar to those in the horse (*see page 16*) may develop in the buccal mucosa of young dogs.

In all three species the majority of neoplasms in the lower alimentary tract are lymphosarcomas (*see page 126*). Adenomas and adeno-carcinomas of the stomach, rectum and rarely the small intestine are found however, most often in the dog, whilst leiomyomas and leiomyosarcomas may also arise from the muscular coats.

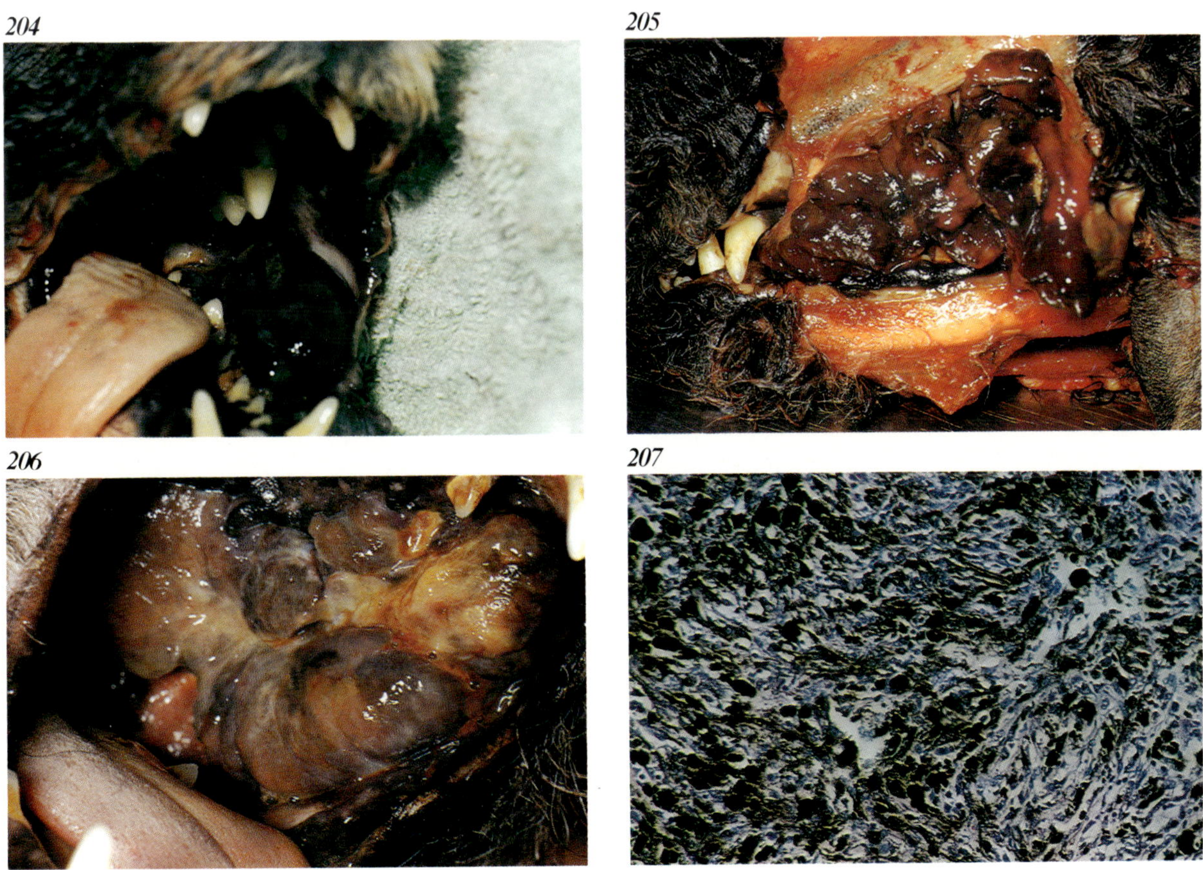

204 *205* *206* *207*

OROPHARYNX

Malignant Melanomas

Occurrence and gross appearance

Malignant melanomas are the most commonly occurring tumours of the mouth in dogs, but are very rare in the horse and cat. In the dog, they originate in the mucous membrane of the lips or gingiva and there is frequently a history of teeth having been extracted before the appearance of a tumour in the gums. Tumours appear as friable, irregularly dome shaped masses with a variable growth rate (***204***). They readily ulcerate and become infected so that the breath becomes foul smelling and bleeding is a frequent complication. They may be obviously darkly pigmented, with a homogeneous, black or dark brown cut surface (***205***), but the less well differentiated tumours are only partly pigmented, or amelanotic (***206***). They are locally very invasive and have no obvious boundaries.

Histological appearance

Melanomas in the mouth are relatively poorly differentiated, being invasive and non-encapsulated. They consist of a homogeneous sheet of polygonal, basophilic cells with a large, pale staining nucleus and indistinct cytoplasmic boundaries. The cells are not normally arranged in a definite architectural pattern but in most tumours, at least some cells will contain dark brown melanin granules (***207***). Occasionally tumours are seen in which no melanin is found, when a definite diagnosis can be difficult to make without employing electron microscopy.

Treatment and prognosis

These tumours are extremely malignant and following surgical removal at least 80% will recur locally, when they sometimes appear to grow more rapidly than the original mass. Widespread metastasis to regional lymph nodes (***208***) and more distant organs is also common. The best form of treatment is radical surgical removal followed by radiotherapy of the local site. Melanomas in the mouth of dogs are frequently radiosensitive and a fractionated dose of 3,000–4,000R, sometimes results in complete remission. Unfortunately, however, most animals treated in this way will die 6–12 months later from multiple lung metastases (***209***).

Squamous Cell Carcinomas

Occurrence and gross appearance

Although squamous cell carcinomas have been described in the oropharynx of all three species they are important only in the cat and dog, particularly in old animals. In cats squamous cell carcinomas are the most commonly occurring tumours of this region, and may be found particularly in the lips, gingiva (***210***), tongue and tonsils, whilst in dogs the gums (***211***), palate and tonsils (***212***) are the usual sites. In all sites these tumours appear as very firm, invasive, fungating, whitish masses with an ulcerated surface and a pale, fibrous, homogeneous cross section. In both dogs and cats squamous cell carcinomas which appear to have originated within the bone of the mandible are sometimes seen (***213***). These tumours cause obvious enlargement and distortion of the lower jaw and can be confused with osteosarcoma on X-ray examination. Squamous cell carcinomas also occur in the oesophagus in cats, where they produce a slowly developing obstruction (***214*** and ***215***).

Histological appearance

This is similar to squamous cell carcinomas in the skin, although tumours tend to be less well differentiated, especially in dogs.

Treatment and prognosis

In cats with intra-oral squamous cell carcinoma the prognosis must always be poor regardless of the site of the tumour or its degree of differentiation. Following surgical intervention most animals will have to be destroyed within three months due to local recurrence, often with regional lymph node or lung metastases being present.

In dogs the prognosis should also be guarded, especially for animals with tonsillar tumours, since these usually recur locally and metastasise readily to the ipsilateral retropharyngeal and anterior cervical lymph nodes and the lungs. Tumours in the gums do not metastasise readily and euthanasia is usually necessary because of the highly erosive and ulcerative nature of these lesions (***216***).

Following surgical removal a significant improvement in survival time will follow X-irradiation of the tumour site, although squamous cell carcinomas appear to be less radio-sensitive than melanomas in the dog.

Fibromas, Fibrosarcomas, and Epulides

Occurrence and gross appearance

This group of tumours is of most importance in dogs and cats. Fibrosarcomas are more common than fibromas in the mouth and they occur more often in the lips or gingiva than in the tongue, palate, or pharynx. They grow relatively slowly but eventually ulcerate through the overlying mucosa and become secondarily infected (***217***). They are firmly attached to, and infiltrate, the underlying tissues, and have a whitish, homogeneous cut surface with a fibrous appearance.

Epulides can occur at any age, and are believed to be derived from the periodontal epithelium. They are usually slowly growing and appear as hard, smooth, pinkish masses, generally less than 2cm in diameter at the gingival border (***218***). In some cases they may be very extensive, occupy most of the gingival margins on both the upper and lower jaws, and may grow around the teeth and obscure them. This type of lesion, which is sometimes referred to as gingival hyperplasia, is most often seen in the Boxer breed. It can also occur in cats (***219***).

The cut surface of the epulis is very hard, and frequently contains irregular spicules of cancellous bone, embedded in a pale, homogeneous fibrous matrix.

Histological appearance

Fibrosarcomas in the mouth are usually fairly well differentiated, and have an identical appearance to those developing in the dermal connective tissues.

Epulides vary considerably in appearance, the commonest form being a relatively acellular and regularly arranged mass of mature connective tissue, covered by an intact,

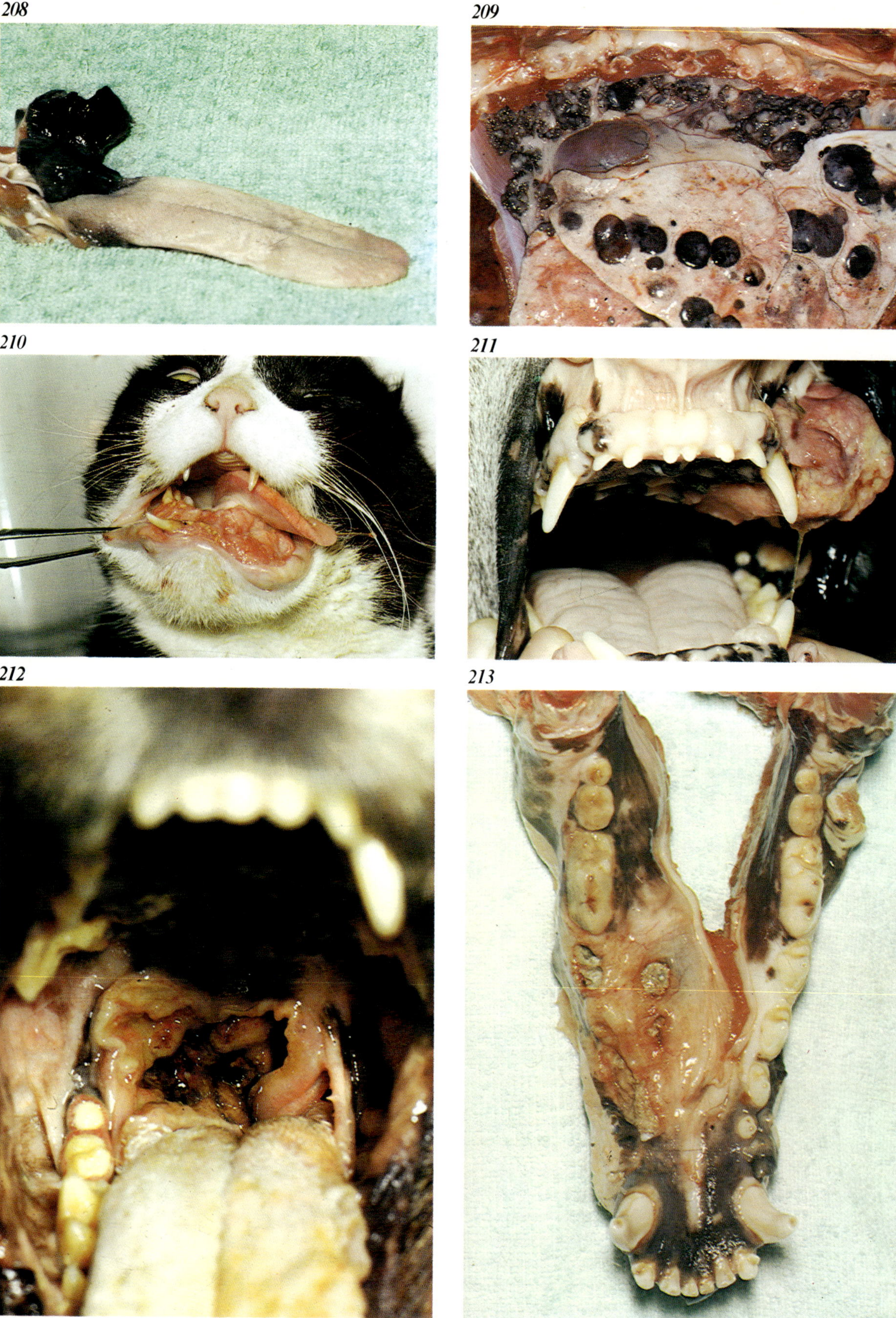
208
209
210
211
212
213

208 *Metastatic lesion in ipsilateral tonsil from a malignant melanoma of the gum – dog.*

209 *Lung metastases from melanoma of the gum in a blue roan Cocker Spaniel.*

210 *Advanced gingival squamous cell carcinoma in the lower jaw of a seven-year-old cat.*

211 *Advanced gingival squamous cell carcinoma – dog.*

212 *Ulcerating tonsillar carcinoma – dog.*

213 *Squamous cell carcinoma arising within the right mandible of a four-year-old Alsatian dog.*

214 *Radiograph of obstruction to the passage of a barium meal in an old cat due to a squamous cell carcinoma of the oesophagus.*

215 *Squamous cell carcinoma of oesophagus – old cat.*

216 *Squamous cell carcinoma of gum with infiltration of the underlying bone. The nasal chamber will eventually be penetrated by the neoplastic process.*

217 *Fibrosarcoma of the lips and gum – cat.*

218 *Typical solitary epulis in a six-year-old Boxer.*

214

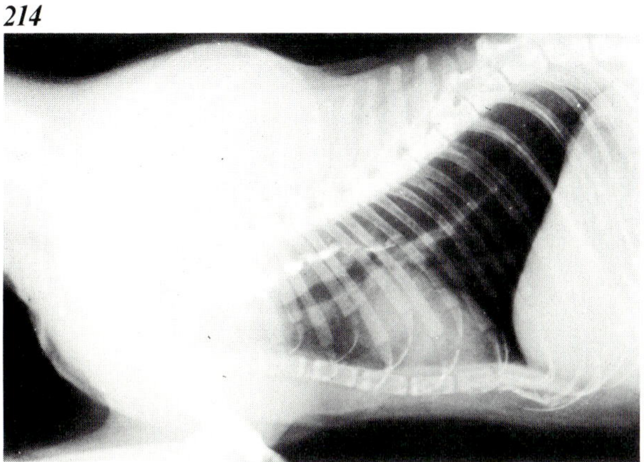

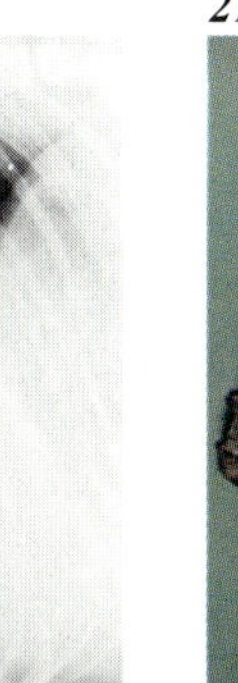

215

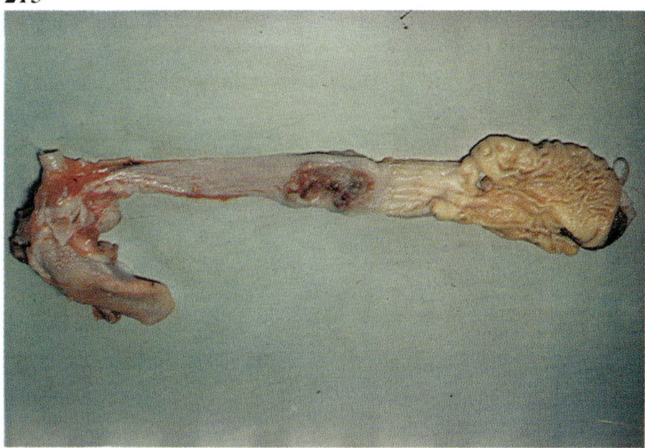

216

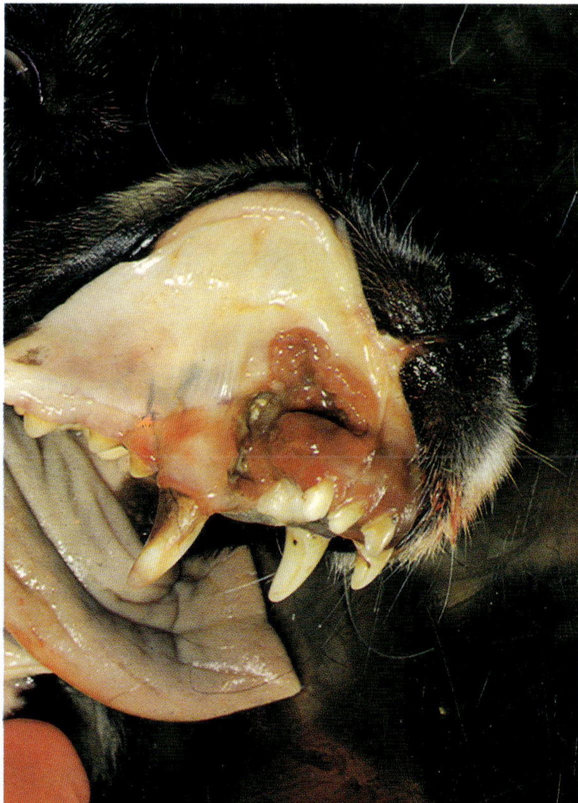

217

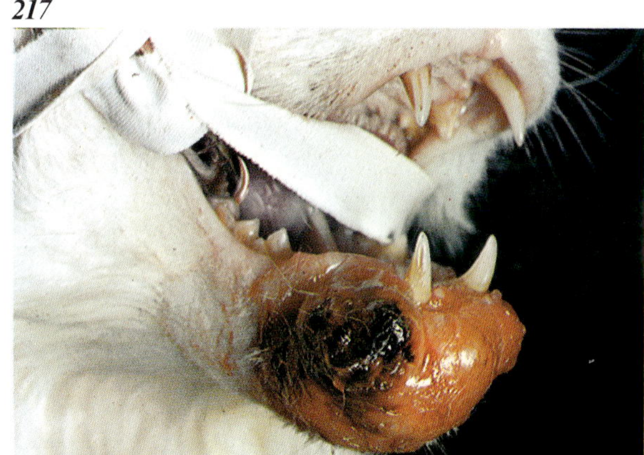

218

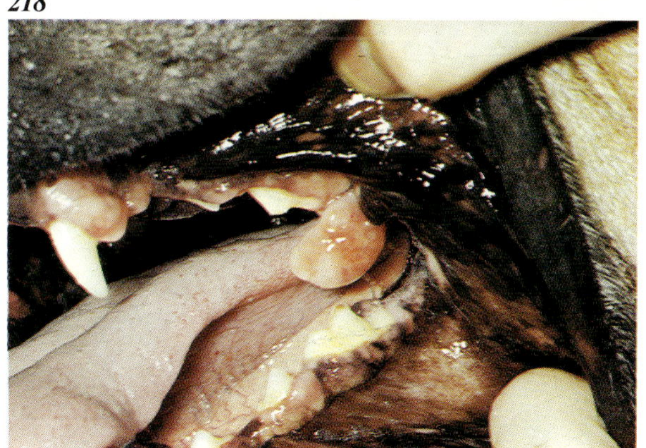

but markedly acanthotic epithelium (*220*), and containing spicules of well calcified osteoid matrix. In some cases, however, the fibrous tissue appears to be extremely active and immature, with long, hyperchromatic spindle shaped cells being arranged in a haphazard fashion within the mass (*221*). In others it is the epithelial elements which are more pronounced, the epithelium sending extremely long, branching rete pegs deep into the mass.

Treatment and prognosis

Single, well differentiated epulides of the classical type carry a favourable prognosis, with surgical removal using diathermy often resulting in a complete cure. In the more active types which nearly always occur in the incisor region in relatively young dogs (*222*) local recurrence is a definite possibility, although metastasis has not been observed. This active type of tumour in young dogs usually grows rapidly and will frequently recur following surgical removal. It may be controlled effectively by the administration of 2,000–3,000R X-irradiation in divided doses following bold surgical excision.

Fibrosarcomas in the mouth, like their counterparts in the skin, do not metastasise at all readily, but are very prone to local recurrence following excision. The prognosis following removal of this type of tumour is poor, especially as they appear to be radio-resistant.

Reticulum Cell Tumours

Occurrence and gross appearance

Reticulum cell tumours in the mouth are confined to dogs, where they usually occur in the lips but are also found in the tongue (*223*). They are rapidly growing and diffusely invasive tumours which may become very large and ulcerate, either through the buccal mucosa or the overlying skin. They have a reddish, usually infected, surface and consist of a soft homogeneous tissue which merges imperceptibly with the surrounding normal tissues. In some cases, instead of forming a single relatively discrete nodule these tumours will produce a diffuse thickening in the connective tissues beneath the mucous membrane of the lips (*224*).

Histological appearance

The histological appearance is similar to that seen in the skin, the lesion consisting of a closely packed sheet of large macrophage-like cells with an indented nucleus, abundant purplish cytoplasm and indistinct cell boundaries. Mitotic figures may be very common and as the cells are not arranged in any definite architectural pattern, they can be confused with poorly differentiated, amelanotic melanomas.

Treatment and prognosis

Because these tumours tend to be diffuse or are very large when first seen, surgical removal is difficult. Even when surgery is possible, local recurrence is common, and the prognosis should always be guarded. Fortunately, however, this type of tumour is very radio-sensitive. Some tumours metastasise to the regional lymph nodes but not usually to more distant organs and it is advisable to either excise the nodes, or to irradiate them at the same time as the primary tumour. Following this form of treatment a number of animals have apparently been cured, although remissions of up to a year are more likely.

Useful palliation may also be achieved by the oral administration of cyclophosphamide (*0.5–2mg/kg*) and prednisolone (*2mg/kg*) every other day.

NON-NEOPLASTIC TUMOUR-LIKE LESIONS OF THE UPPER ALIMENTARY TRACT

Granulomas

Occurrence and gross appearance

In cats, eosinophilic granulomas may be seen on the margins or inside of the lips (*225*), at the base of the external nares, or on the tongue, where they appear as deep, roughly circular ulcers up to 1cm in diameter (*227*). They can be confused with invasive squamous cell carcinomas in these sites. Granulomas may also be seen in the mucous membranes of the angles of the jaws, where they are almost always bilateral and tend to extend forward along the tooth margins (*226*). These granulomas are nodular and have a fleshy, pinkish appearance. They may ulcerate through the mucosa, bleed, or become secondarily infected and interfere with feeding.

Histological appearance

The superficial areas of eosinophilic granulomas are heavily secondarily infected, whilst the dermal connective tissues are infiltrated by large numbers of eosinophil polymorphs, amongst which macrophages, plasma cells, and lymphocytes are scattered.

Granulomas at the angles of the jaws are somewhat similar in appearance but eosinophils are not conspicuous and macrophages and plasma cells are the predominant cell types.

Aetiology

The cause of these lesions is unknown, but it has been suggested that they may be of viral aetiology. An alternative theory is that eosinophilic granulomas arise as a result of continual licking of the site following mild trauma.

Treatment and prognosis

Eosinophilic granulomas are best treated by surgical removal where this is possible. An arrest of the erosion can sometimes follow painting with gentian violet (1%) with or without broad spectrum antibiotics. In the larger lesions radiotherapy up to a total dose of 1,500R may be of benefit.

Granulomatous lesions in the mouth itself are often very difficult to treat but prolonged administration of corticosteroids and tetracyclines may achieve useful remissions.

Dentigerous Cysts

Occurrence and gross appearance

Dentigerous cysts, which arise from the enamel organ after the completion of amelogenesis, are seen in dogs and horses, mostly occurring in young animals during the

219 *Multiple epulides (gingival hyperplasia) in a young Siamese cat.*

220 *Epulis – dog. Note the proliferation of the covering epithelium. H & E.*

221 *More active epulis with rapid proliferation of the stromal fibroblasts. H & E.*

222 *Active epulis in the lower gum of a four-year-old yellow Labrador. This fungating type of lesion is expecially prone to local recurrence.*

223 *Reticulum cell sarcoma beneath the tongue of a nine-year-old Labrador.*

224 *Reticulum cell sarcoma in the upper lip of a Boxer. The tumour is only slightly raised above the surrounding mucosa and has an indistinct edge.*

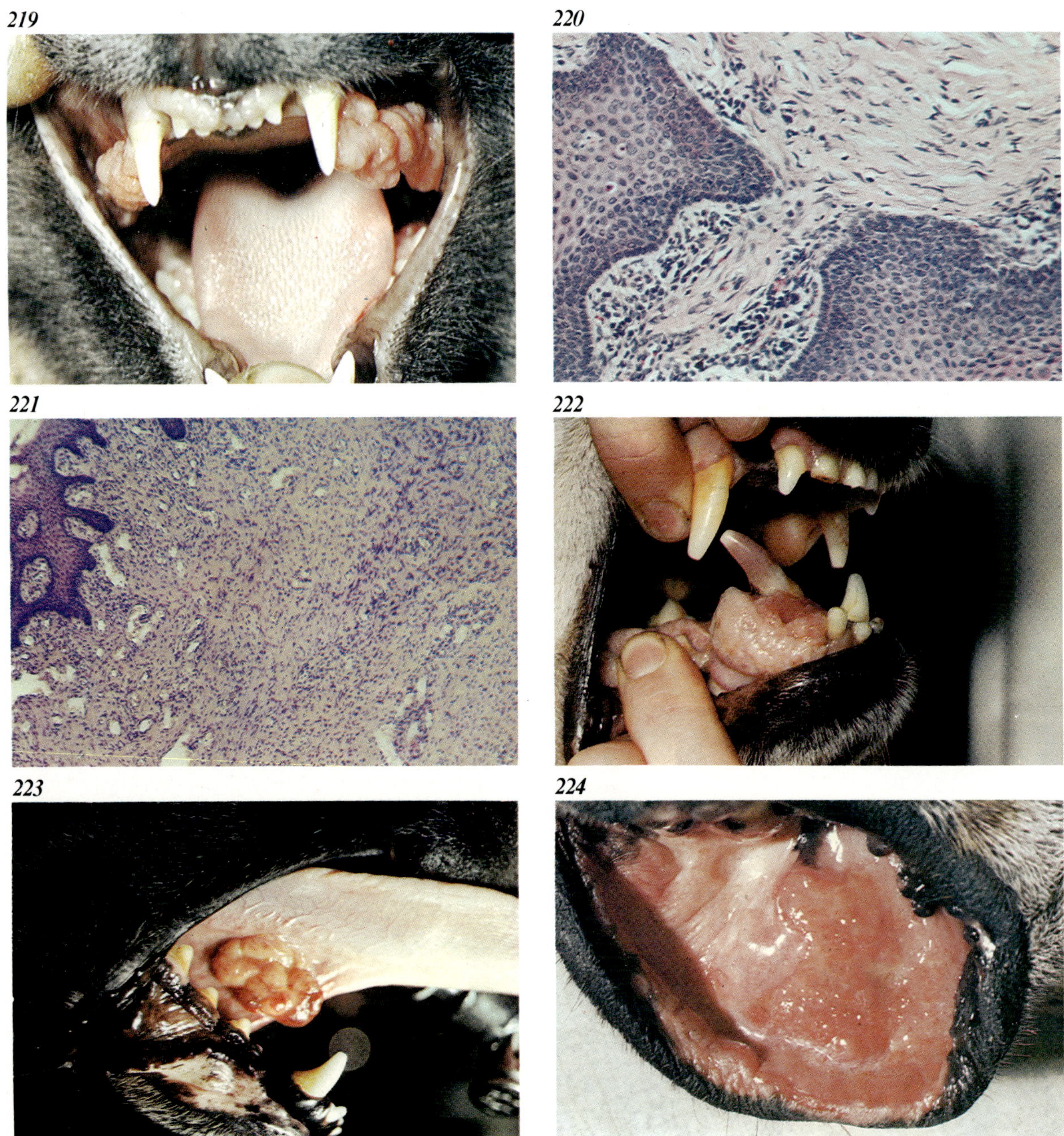

225 *Eosinophilic granuloma (rodent ulcer) in upper lip of cat.*

226 *Granulomas at angle of jaw – cat. These lesions are usually bilateral. There is also evidence of gingivitis in this case.*

227 *Eosinophilic granuloma on tongue – cat.*

228 *Dentigerous cyst in parotid region – two-year-old gelding.*

229 *Single large tooth embedded in petrous temporal bone, dentigerous cyst – horse.*

230 *Fibrosarcoma induced by Spirocerca lupi in the oesophagus of a dog. Smaller granulomas containing parasites are also apparent.*

225

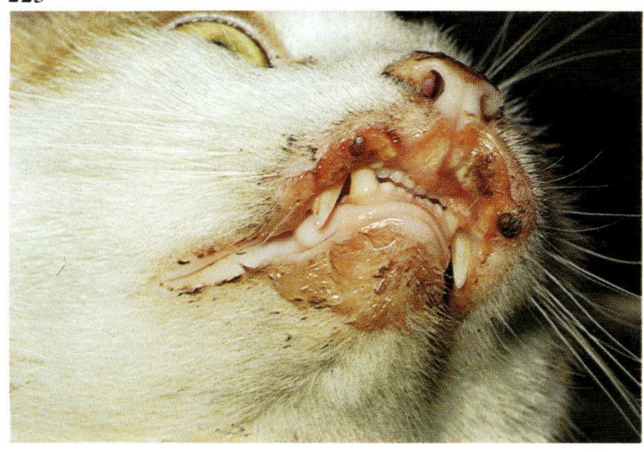

226

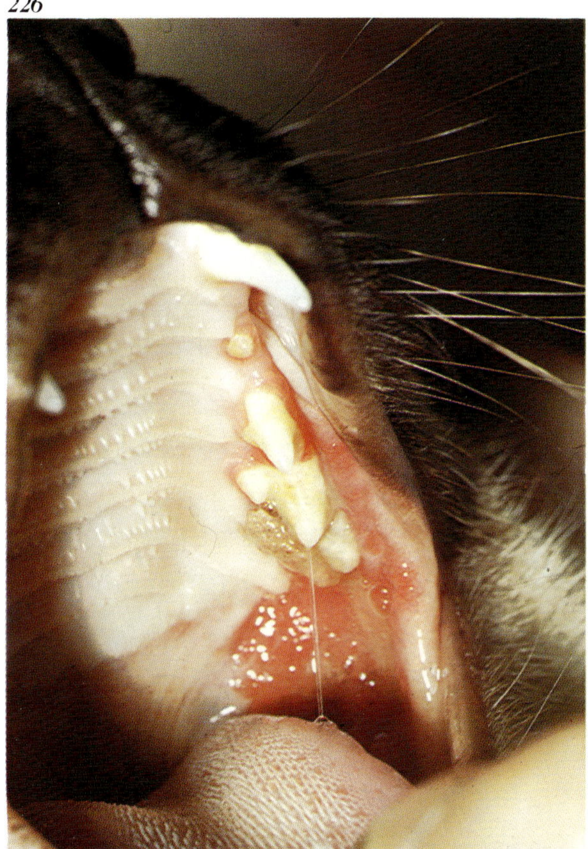

227

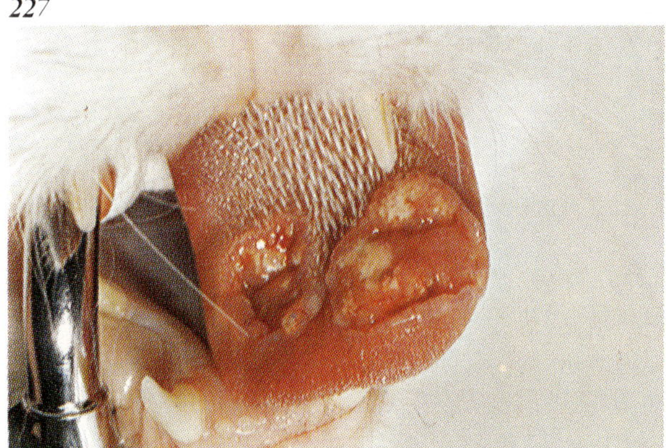

228

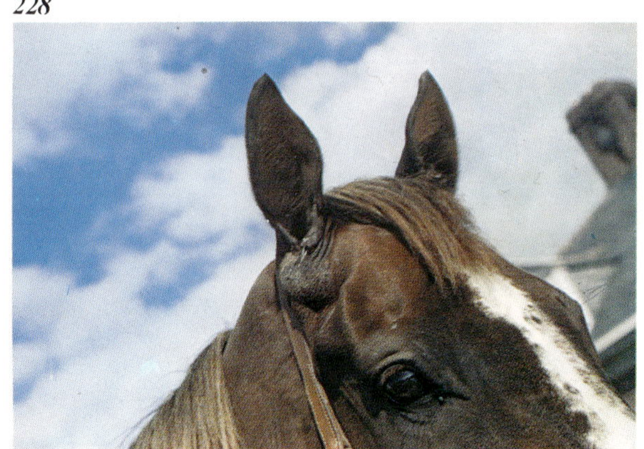

229

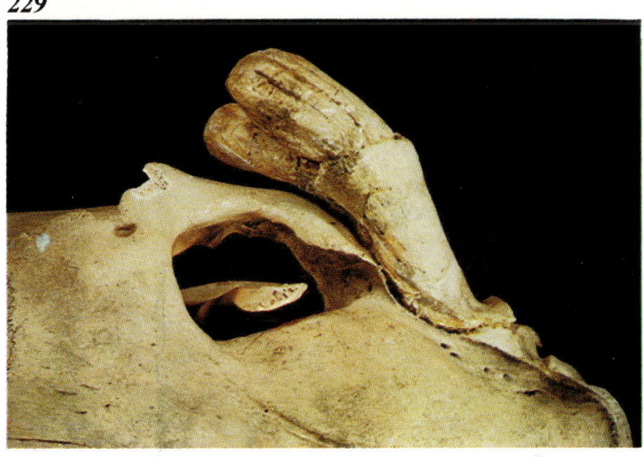

230

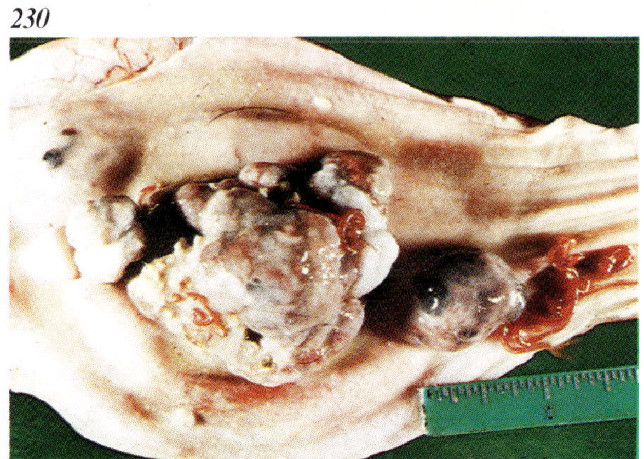

period when there is active tooth development. In horses these lesions present as a fluctuating, apparently cystic mass near the base of the ear (*228*). The cyst increases in size and eventually ruptures through the skin, releasing a clear, gelatinous fluid. The cyst is lined by a smooth membrane and usually contains a single tooth, which may be embedded in the petrous temporal bone (*229*) or be found lying freely in the lumen. Occasionally multiple teeth may be present within the cyst. In the dog cysts containing one or more teeth occur adjacent to the normal teeth in the mouth.

Histological appearance

The cyst wall is composed of a fibrous capsule lined by stratified squamous epithelium.

Treatment and prognosis

The prognosis is good following complete surgical excision of the cyst lining, but if a portion of the wall is left in situ a sinus persists.

Lesions Associated with Spirocerca Lupi in Dogs

Occurrence and gross appearance

Spirocerca lupi is a nematode which is parasitic in the dog, fox, and wolf, where it inhabits the walls of the oesophagus, stomach, and aorta. It is relatively common in most sub-tropical and tropical areas. The lesions in the oesophagus, originally small and symptomless, grow into large nodular masses with a pale, firm cut surface and in some animals sarcomatous transformation occurs (*230*).

Histological appearance

Early lesions appear as granulomas. Tumours usually have the typical appearance of fibrosarcomas, similar to those seen in the skin and other organs, although osteosarcomas have also been described.

Aetiology

Although these neoplasms are obviously related to *S. lupi* infestation, the underlying cause of the malignant transformation is obscure.

Treatment and prognosis

The prognosis for dogs in which malignant transformation has occurred is very poor since in more than half these cases there is metastasis to the lungs. Many dogs develop pulmonary osteoarthropathy (*Marie's disease*).

TUMOURS OF THE STOMACH AND INTESTINES

Adenomas and Adenocarcinomas

Occurrence and gross appearance

Adenomas or 'polyps' are seen most commonly in the dog, where they can occur at any site, but are seen mainly in the pyloric area of the stomach, the duodenum, and the last few centimetres of the rectum. In the stomach or duodenum they manifest themselves clinically by causing vomiting a few hours after feeding, while in the terminal rectum they give rise to straining and the passage of blood-stained faeces. Diagnosis may require X-ray examination following administration of a barium meal, or an exploratory laparotomy. These tumours are usually fairly small, firm, pedunculated lesions which are attached to the mucosa by a narrow pedicle. They have a pale, fibrous cut surface and are covered by numerous, small, thin, papillary structures, giving the whole mass a velvety appearance (*231*). There is no evidence of infiltration into the underlying connective tissues and the pedicle is freely mobile over the muscular coats.

Adenocarcinomas are not common in any species. In dogs they are found most frequently in the stomach and rectum, where they produce clinical signs similar to those produced by adenomas. They appear grossly as very poorly circumscribed, irregular, thickened areas in the wall, which in the case of the stomach may involve almost the whole of the organ (*232*). The mucosa overlying the lesion becomes ulcerated and secondarily infected while the affected area of the wall is very firm in consistency and has a whitish homogeneous cut surface which completely replaces the normal musculature. Large, multinodular carcinomas may also develop in the small intestine, where they cause partial or complete obstruction (*233 and 234*).

Histological appearance

Adenomas consist of a central stalk of dense connective tissue which is covered by tall columnar epithelial cells forming branching papillae or acinar structures (*235*). Many cells contain droplets of mucin but there is no evidence of infiltration of the connective tissues by epithelial cells.

Adenocarcinomas vary considerably in their degree of differentiation; rectal lesions usually being well differentiated compared to those in the stomach. Well differentiated tumours consist of a dense fibrous stroma containing irregularly shaped, often cystic, acini lined by a single layer of epithelial cells containing large droplets of mucin (*236*). The lumen of the acini also contains a mucinous secretion. Even well differentiated tumours are invasive and neoplastic structures can be seen throughout the wall of the organ. Poorly differentiated tumours, as seen in the stomach, consist of large epithelial cells which are diffusely invading the wall of the organ. The cells do not usually form recognisable glandular structures (*237*) but frequently contain intracytoplasmic droplets of mucin which can be seen with special staining techniques (*238*), giving the cells a characteristic 'signet ring' appearance.

Treatment and prognosis

The prognosis following surgical removal of adenomas should be favourable, although local recurrence can still present problems, especially with rectal polyps. Following the

231 *Large polyp being excised surgically.*

233 *Radiograph of obstruction to the passage of barium by a carcinoma of the small intestine in an 11-year-old Alsation bitch. The barium had been administered orally five hours previously.*

234 *Adenocarcinoma of the proximal duodenum – horse.*

232 *Diffuse thickening of the stomach wall by a poorly differentiated gastric adenocarcinoma. So called 'leather bottle' stomach.*

235 *Well differentiated gastric 'polyp' – dog. There is no invasion of the underlying stroma by epithelial cells. H & E.*

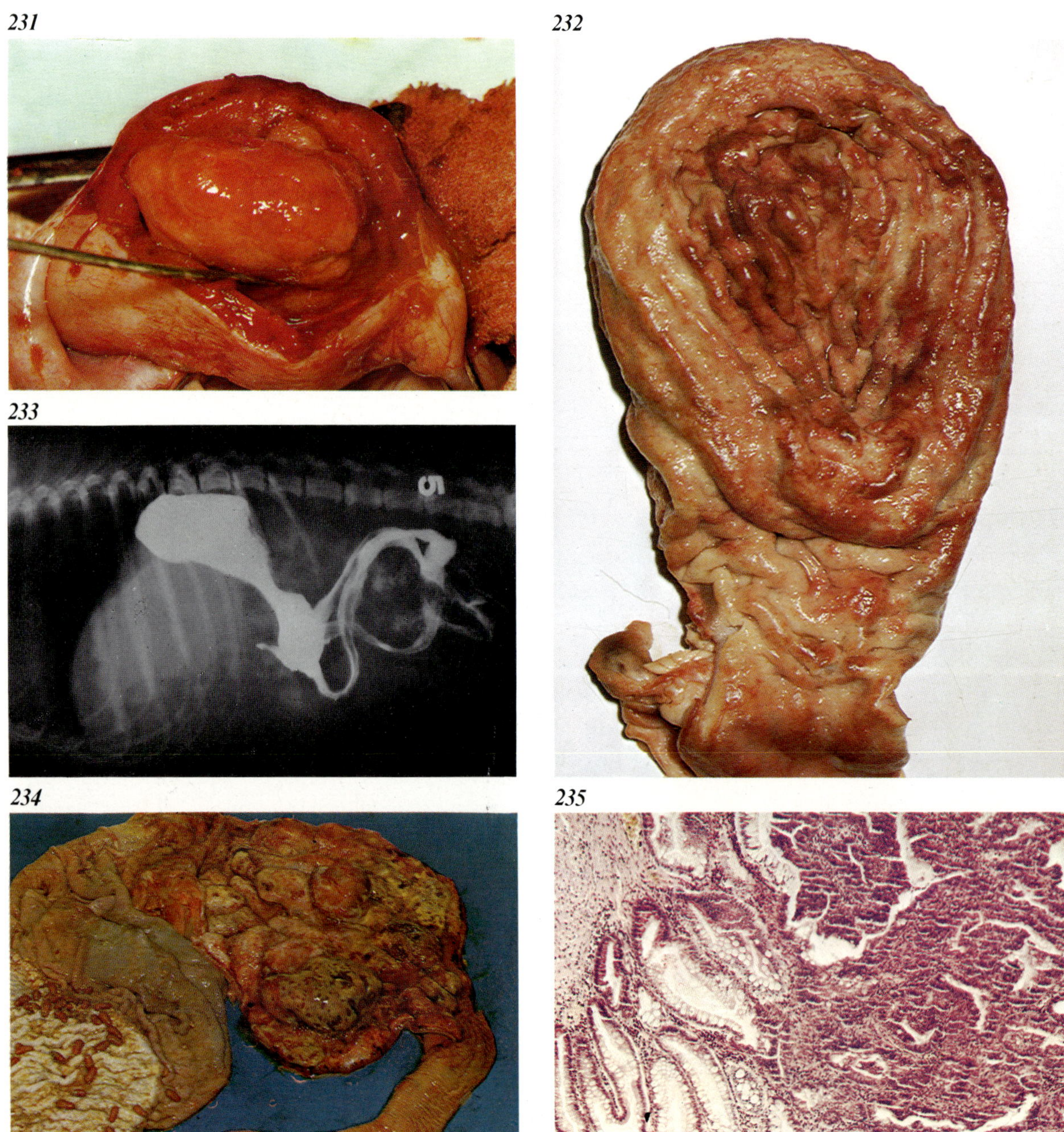

236 *Well differentiated rectal adenocarcinoma. Masson's trichrome.*

237 *Poorly differentiated adenocarcinoma of the gastric mucosa in a dog. The cells are not forming glandular structures but many contain a single large globule of mucus. These are known as 'signet ring' cells. H & E.*

238 *Vascular invasion by a poorly differentiated gastric carcinoma – Alcian blue stain.*

239 *Trans-abdominal (mesenteric) and haematogenous (hepatic) metastases from an intestinal adenocarcinoma – cat.*

240 *Adenocarcinoma of terminal rectum – dog. Note the annular appearance of these tumours.*

236

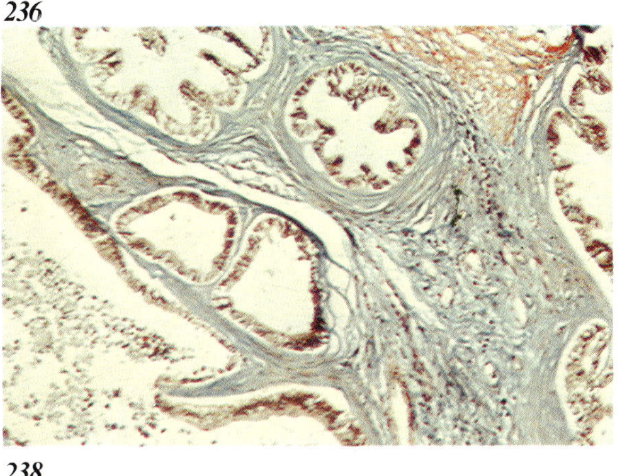

237

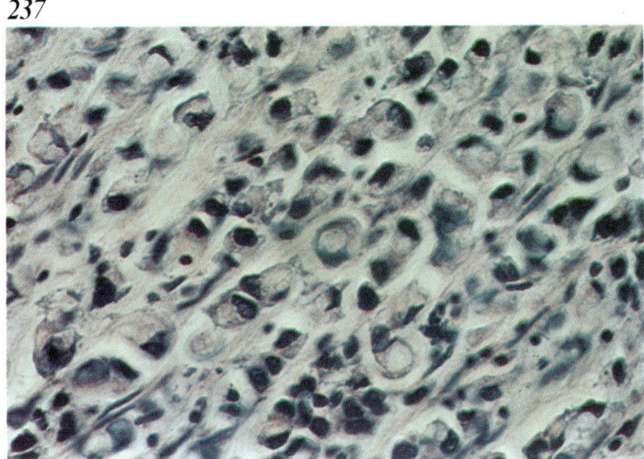

238

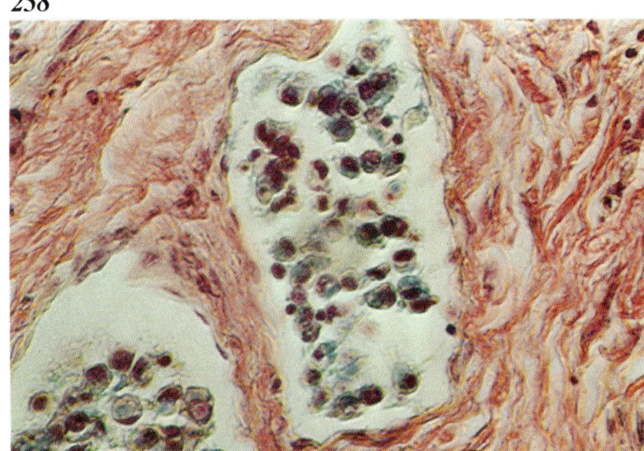

239

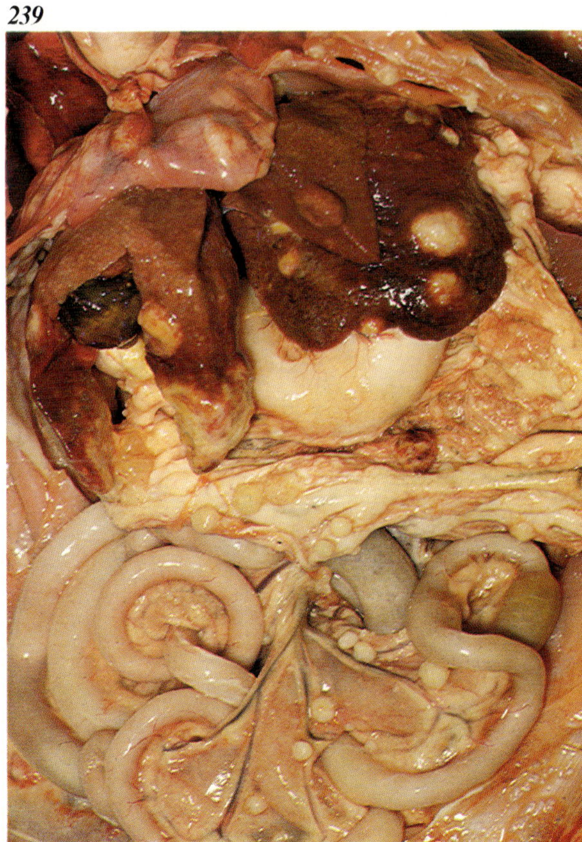

240

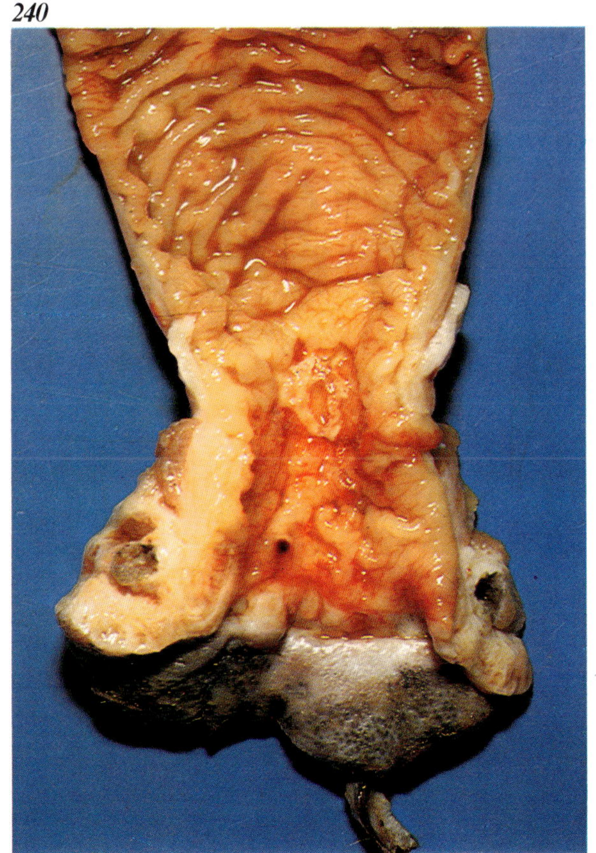

surgical excision of adenocarcinomas the prognosis is poor, with transabdominal and haematogenous metastasis being common (***239***).

Rectal carcinomas often produce a constriction of the lumen a few centimetres anterior to the anal sphincter (***240***). If a cruciate incision is made at this site extending as far as the serosa followed by the daily insertion of a dilator to prevent further constrictive healing, the immediate results are beneficial. Straining ceases and as the tumour is slow growing the animal may live a normal life for a further few months. Early radical excision of low grade rectal carcinoma can result in long term remission.

Chapter 10
The Liver and Pancreas

Bile Duct Carcinomas

Occurrence and gross appearance

Tumours of the bile ducts occur most frequently in dogs where they account for most primary hepatic neoplasms, but have also been described in cats and horses. They are almost always multiple and since clinical manifestations appear late in the course of the disease, are often extremely large when first diagnosed. Clinical signs include abdominal distension, pain, inappetence and severe ascites, the abdomen sometimes containing a large volume of blood-stained fluid. Examination of the affected liver usually reveals one or more lobes to have been entirely replaced by a large, irregularly shaped, yellowish-white mass, with a rather friable cut surface mottled by areas of haemorrhage and necrosis.

There are frequently multiple smaller tumours scattered throughout the hepatic parenchyma, these lesions being well circumscribed, roughly spherical, and measuring up to several centimetres in diameter (***241***).

Because of the multiple nature of bile duct carcinomas it is often difficult to differentiate them from hepatic metastases from other intra-abdominal tumours. Thus before a diagnosis of bile duct carcinoma is made, the possibility of other primary tumours must be investigated.

Histological appearance

Well differentiated tumours are composed of large cystic acinar structures, lined by a single layer of columnar epithelial cells (***242***).

Poorly differentiated tumours are usually more invasive, and are composed of much smaller, irregular acini, lined by very hyperchromatic, pleomorphic cells (***243***).

Treatment and prognosis

The prognosis is always poor as nearly all animals with this type of tumour show intra-hepatic metastases when seen. Pulmonary metastases are also common.

Hepatomas and Hepatic Carcinomas

Occurrence and gross appearance

Hepatomas are seen most often in dogs, where they may be more common than has been previously supposed. They are rare tumours in the horse and cat.

When hepatomas are first diagnosed they are generally very large since they produce few clinical signs in the early stages. They manifest themselves by abdominal swelling, inappetence, and sometimes vomiting, these signs usually developing rapidly. Abdominal palpation reveals a very large intra-abdominal mass and radiography is helpful in diagnosis.

Definite diagnosis can be made by exploratory laparotomy, when the liver is seen to contain a large, usually solitary mass many centimetres in diameter. The tumour generally has a very broad base (***244***), but can be pedunculated and attached to the remainder of the liver by a thin stalk (***245***). It is irregular in shape and has a yellowish-brown cut surface which may contain areas of haemorrhage and necrosis.

Histological appearance

These tumours are composed of well differentiated hepatocytes and it is difficult to distinguish between benign and malignant types histologically. The hepatocytes are usually arranged in solid lobules (***246***), although they sometimes are seen lining blood-filled sinusoids as in the normal liver.

There is no evidence of normal hepatic lobulation in the tumour so that definite portal triads and central veins are lacking and for this reason many cells show obvious fatty infiltration (***247***).

241 *Multiple bile duct adenocarcinomas – cat.*

242 *Well differentiated bile duct adenocarcinoma – dog. H & E.*

243 *Poorly differentiated bile duct adenocarcinoma – dog. H & E.*

244 *Broad based, solitary hepatoma – dog.*

241

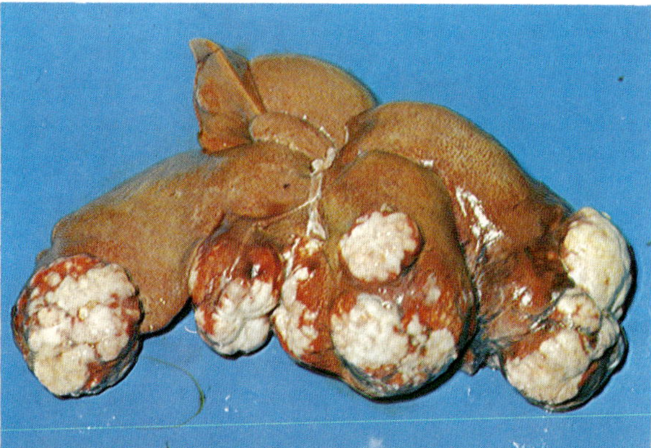

242

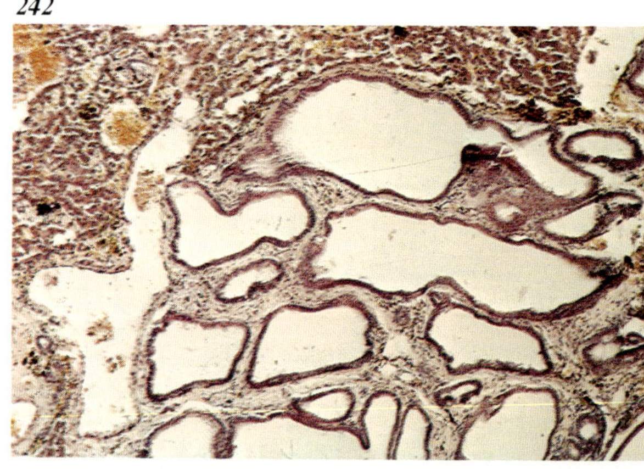

243

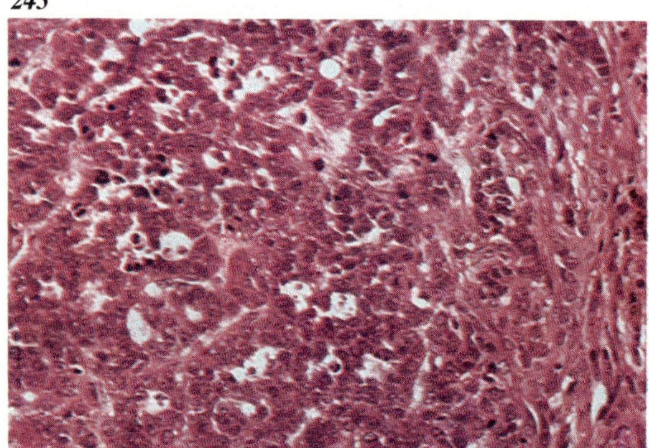

244

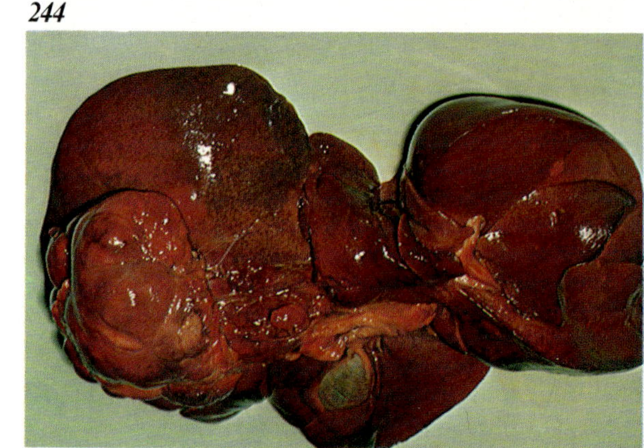

Treatment and prognosis

The prognosis is poor. In some cases the animal dies suddenly due to rupture of the capsule of the liver followed by massive intra-abdominal haemorrhage.

Surgical removal of the affected lobe is sometimes possible and has resulted in cures but more often the animal later dies from regional lymph node or lung metastases.

---

245 *Pedunculated hepatoma – dog.*

246 *Hepatoma – dog. The cells are arranged in small solid clumps and have vacuolated cytoplasm. H & E.*

247 *Hepatoma stained for fat. Many cells apparently contain little else. Oil red O.*

248 *Benign nodular hyperplasia of the liver – dog.*

249 *Bovine tuberculosis affecting the liver and spleen of a horse. This animal had been grazing with a herd of tuberculous cattle.*

250 *Tuberculous granuloma – horse. Note the relative absence of necrosis, the abundant fibrous reaction and the Langhan's-type giant cells. Masson's trichrome.*

245

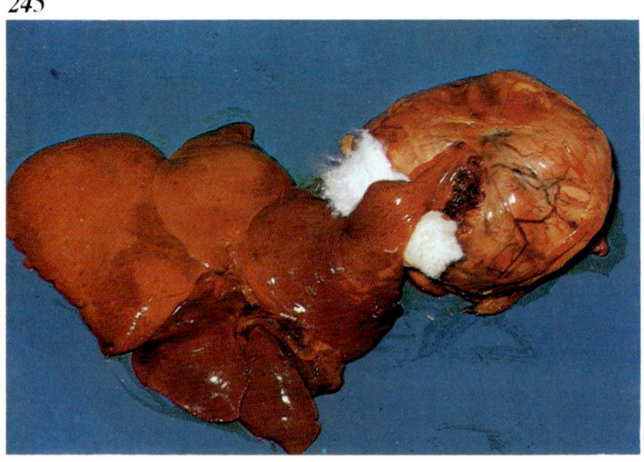

246

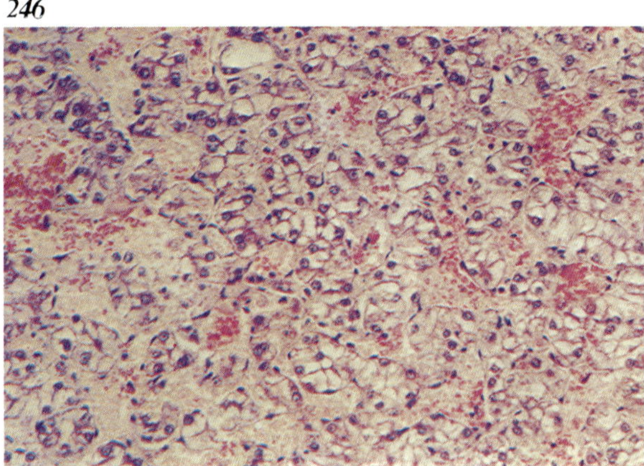

247

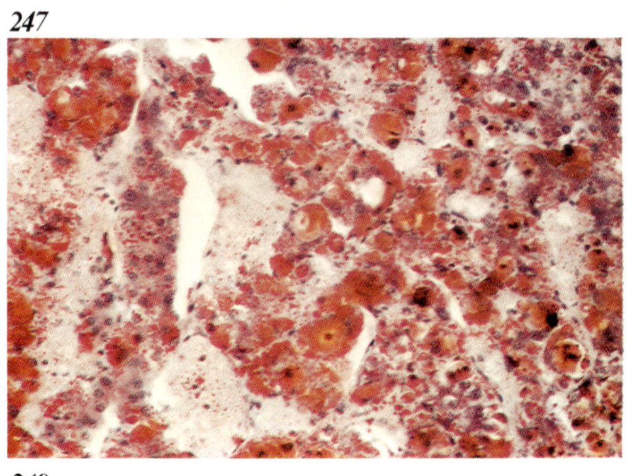

248

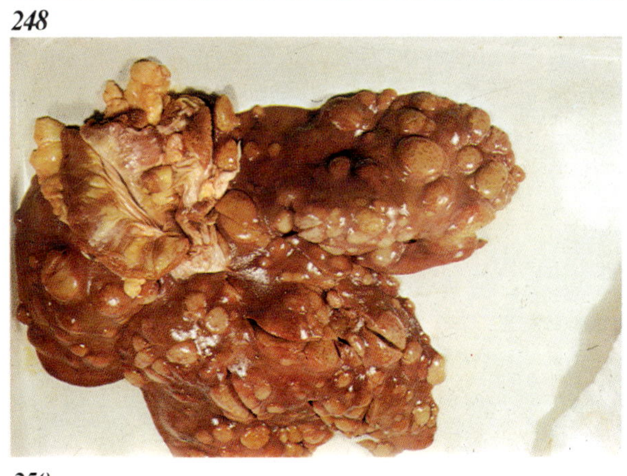

249

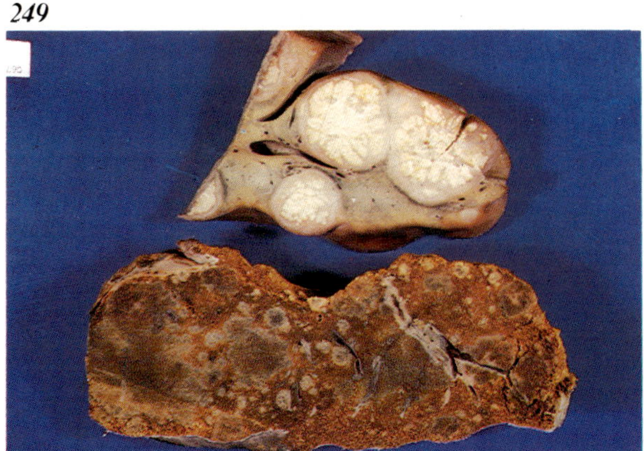

250

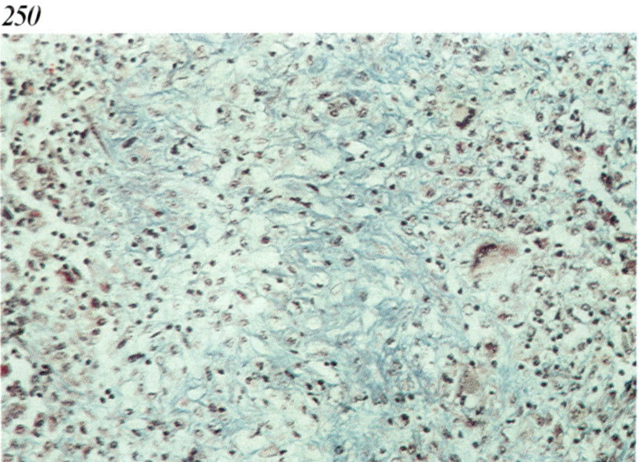

NON-NEOPLASTIC TUMOUR-LIKE LESIONS AFFECTING THE LIVER

Benign Nodular Hyperplasia of the Liver

Occurrence and gross appearance

This condition, which affects only the dog, is seen in middle-aged or older animals. The liver is irregular in shape, the surface being distorted by numerous spherical, yellowish or red nodules varying in size from 1–3cm or more in diameter (***248***). The cut surface of the nodules is homogeneous, yellowish-brown or red in colour and rather greasy or friable in texture. The nodules are separated from each other by apparently normal liver parenchyma, and it is usually difficult to determine where the lesion ends and normal parenchyma begins.

Histological appearance

The histological appearance is similar to that seen in hepatomas, although the multiple nature of these lesions, and their relatively small size help to distinguish them from true tumours.

Treatment and prognosis

Once signs develop the prognosis is very poor. No medical treatment is known for this condition, and the multiple nature of the lesions renders surgical intervention impossible. Sudden death may occur due to rupture of the capsule and massive intra-abdominal haemorrhage, or due to the proliferation of clostridia in the anoxic centre of the larger lesions.

Hepatic Tuberculosis

Occurrence and gross appearance

Although hepatic tuberculosis may be seen in any of the three species it is only likely to be confused with neoplasia in the horse. The tumour-like lesions appear in the liver and spleen as firm, well circumscribed, whitish masses up to several centimetres in diameter (***249***). Their cut surface has an obviously fibrous appearance but this usually contains a number of tiny foci of yellowish necrosis. Similar lesions are also present in the mesenteric lymph nodes. The histological appearance is typical of a granulomatous inflammatory reaction (***250***) but acid fast organisms are usually difficult to find.

TUMOURS OF THE PANCREAS

Adenomas and Adenocarcinomas of the Exocrine Gland

Occurrence and gross appearance

Small, multiple pancreatic adenomas, virtually indistinguishable from hyperplastic nodules, are common incidental findings in old dogs on post mortem examination, but are of little clinical significance.

Pancreatic carcinomas are among the commonest intra-abdominal tumours in the dog and are also seen in cats. They are usually manifested clinically by lethargy, inappetence, and sometimes, abdominal swelling, with some animals developing obstructive jaundice due to pressure on the common bile duct where it enters the duodenum (*251*). Radiographs may reveal an intra-abdominal mass, but it is frequently necessary to perform an exploratory laparotomy to make a definite diagnosis. Gross examination reveals the presence of a large, very firm, multinodular mass which has completely replaced one limb of the pancreas and which is closely adherent to the omentum and surrounding tissues (*252*). The cut surface of the tumour is pale in colour, firm and homogeneous, although large tumours may contain zones of necrosis.

Histological appearance

The degree of differentiation of these tumours is variable but many are composed of regular acini with a small central lumen surrounded by tall, columnar cells (*253*). Poorly differentiated tumours composed of solid foci of hyperchromatic cells are also common.

Treatment and prognosis

The prognosis is always very poor as most tumours have already metastasised to the liver, and less commonly the spleen and kidneys, when they are first diagnosed.

Tumours of the Pancreatic Islets

Occurrence and gross appearance

These are rare tumours of the dog and cat but are of interest because of their ability to produce insulin in some cases. Animals with insulin producing tumours exhibit periodic bouts of hypoglycaemia, manifested by convulsions, loss of consciousness, ataxia and weakness. Blood glucose levels are low and there is a dramatic response to glucose given intravenously. The primary tumour is frequently small, but much larger tumours are seen on occasion and may be multiple. The tumours are characteristically yellowish-brown in colour and firm in consistency.

Histological appearance

These tumours consist of numerous relatively small, solid lobules of neoplastic epithelial cells (*254*) or cells arranged as irregularly shaped, thin walled acini with a large lumen. The cells have a central, spherical, hyperchromatic nucleus and a variable amount of granular cytoplasm. There is sometimes evidence of 'palisading' of cells at the edge of the lobule. The cytoplasm of beta cells stains purple with Gomori's aldehyde fuchsin stain.

Treatment and prognosis

The dramatic clinical signs may lead to an early diagnosis in these malignant tumours. Surgical excision can result in a complete cure but the operation itself carries a high risk of acute pancreatic necrosis. In those cases where metastases are seen at laparotomy, the prognosis is hopeless.

251 *Obstruction to the common bile duct by a pancreatic adenocarcinoma – dog.*

252 *Pancreatic adenocarcinoma with metastasis to the liver – dog.*

253 *Secondary pancreatic adenocarcinoma in the liver. The well formed acini closely resemble those of the normal pancreas. H & E.*

254 *Islet cell tumour – dog. Gomori's aldehyde fuchsin.*

251

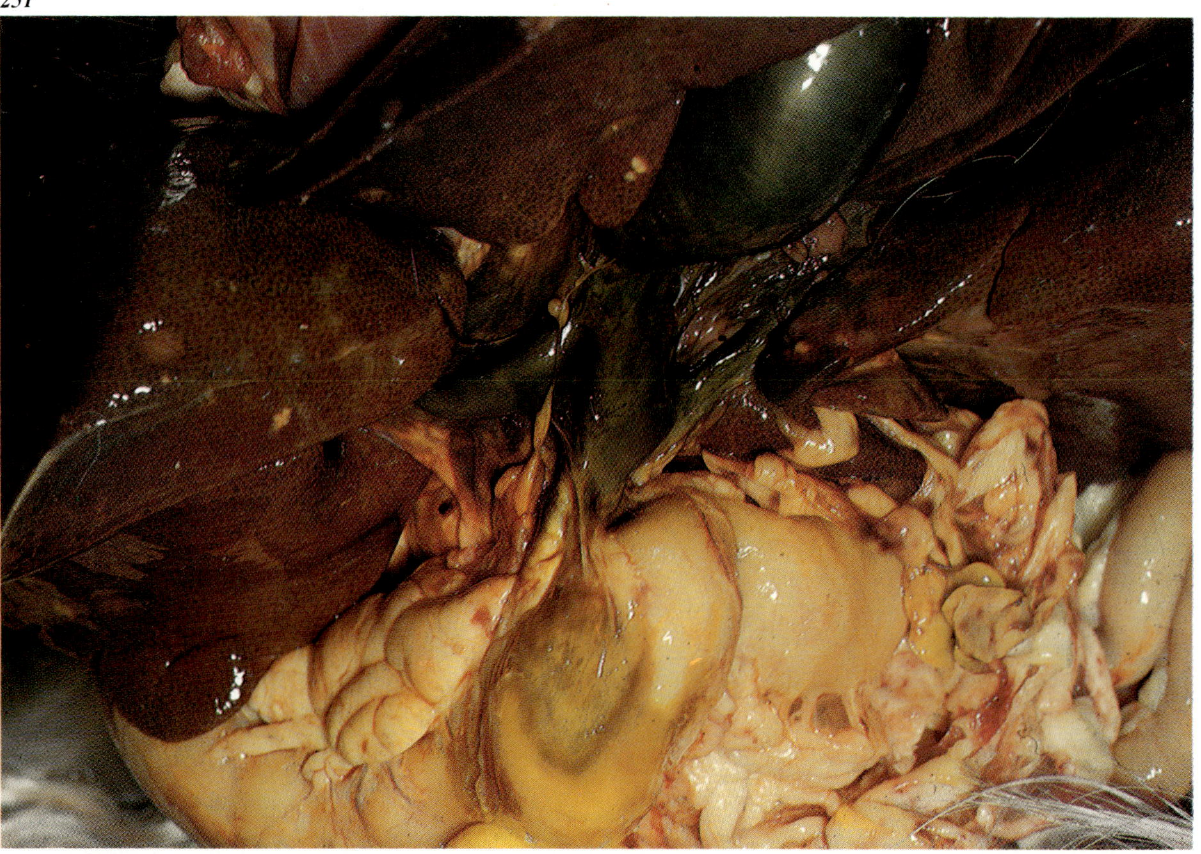

252

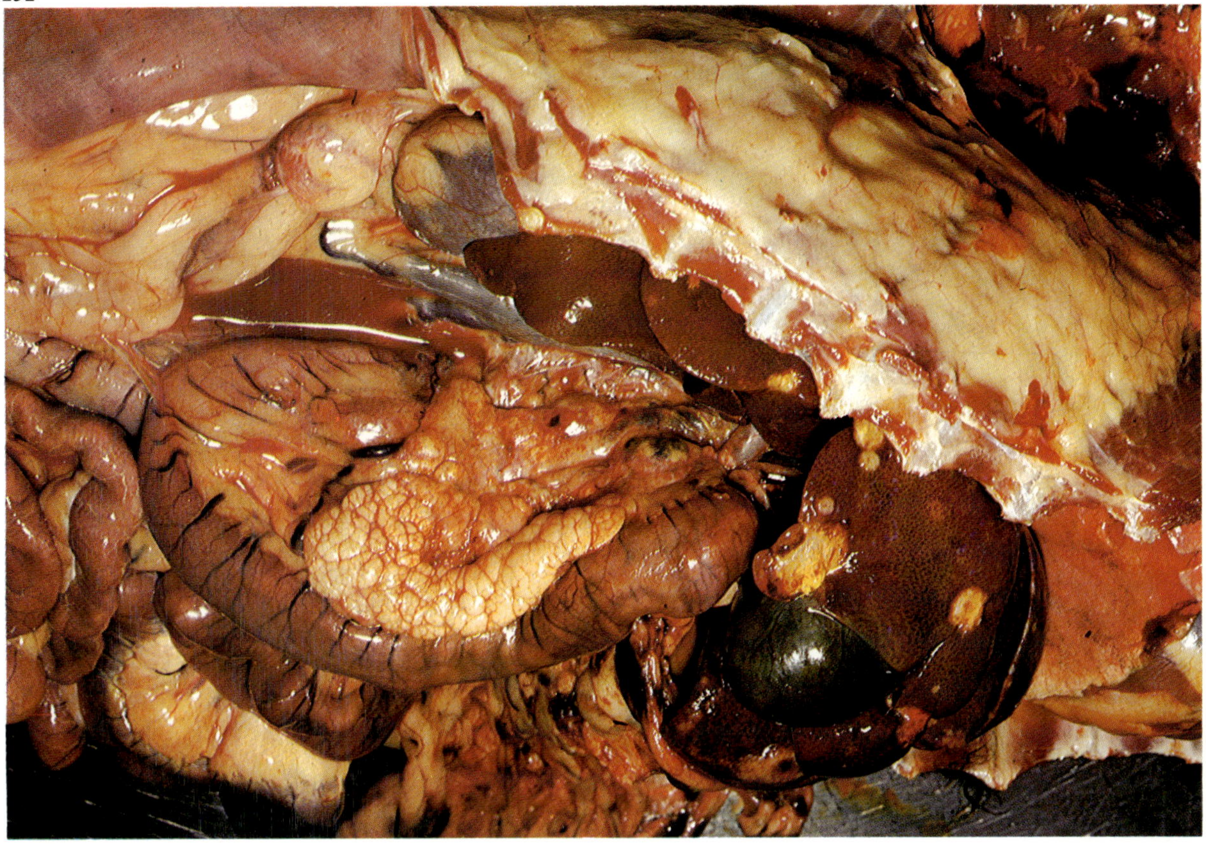

253

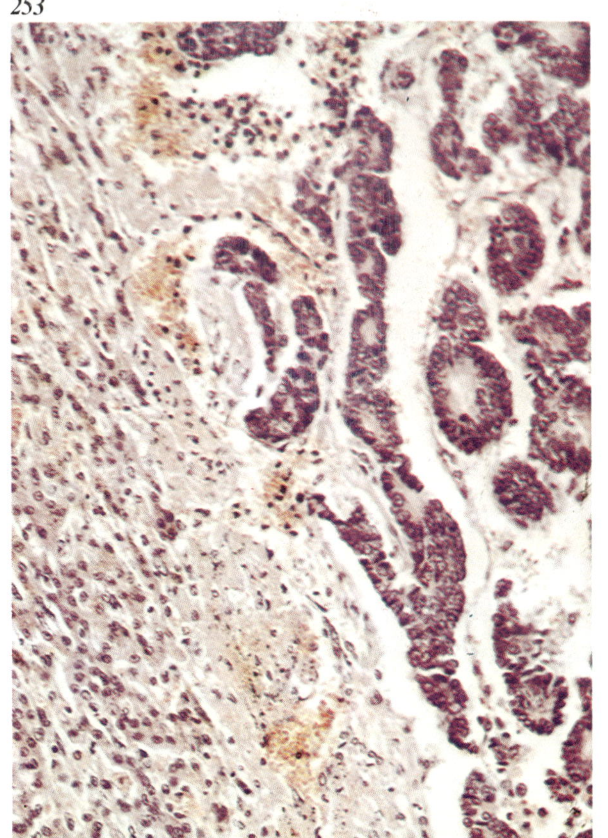

254

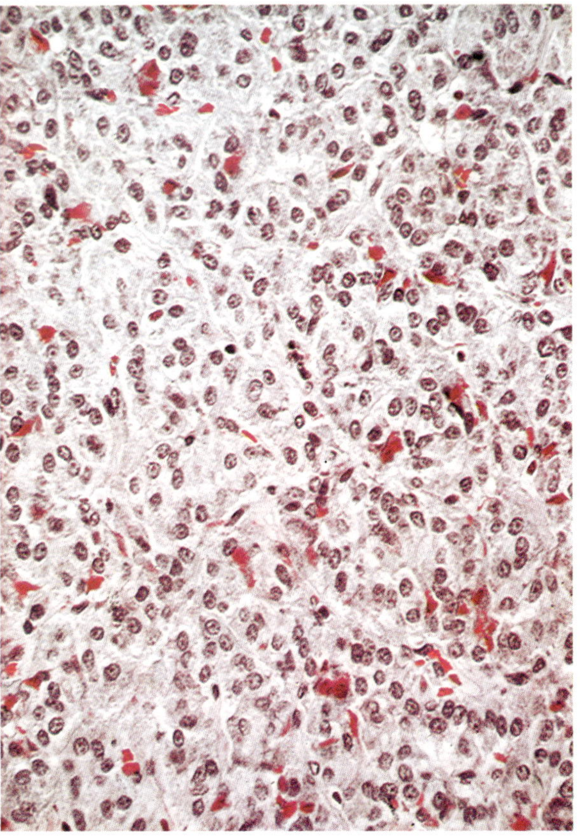

Chapter 11
The Lymphoid and Vascular Tissue

Solid lymphoid neoplasms are very much commoner than leukaemias in animals and have been given a variety of names, including malignant lymphoma, leukosis, lymphocytoma, pseudo-Hodgkin's disease and lymphosarcoma. The last is now in general usage and is preferred.

Lymphosarcomas

Occurrence and gross appearance

Lymphosarcoma is the most common neoplasm in cats, is also very common in dogs, but is unusual in horses. There are a number of fairly distinct anatomical types of lymphosarcoma although there is some overlap between them, with multicentric, alimentary and thymic types being the commonest.

Most cases in dogs occur in animals over four years of age, the majority being of the multicentric type, although alimentary and thymic types are also seen. The main clinical features in the first type are bilateral enlargement of the peripheral lymph nodes and tonsils, with hepatosplenomegaly (***255** and **256***). Infiltration of the anterior chamber of the eye with lymphocytes is sometimes seen, although this feature is commoner in cats (***257***), and anaemia is usually present. Gross examination of affected lymph nodes reveals them to be enlarged, well circumscribed and firm, with a whitish, homogeneous, oedematous and bulging cut surface (***258***). There is a complete loss of differentiation between cortex and medulla and in advanced cases the nodes may be necrotic and partially liquefied. Sometimes defined nodules of tumour are visible in the liver, spleen, heart and lungs.

In cats the alimentary and thymic types are the most common, the multicentric type being rather unusual. Clinical signs in the alimentary type include severe diarrhoea or dysentery, often accompanied by anorexia and vomiting. A sausage shaped mass of tumorous intestine resembling an intussusception may be palpable but in some cases infiltration is more extensive and diffuse. The small intestine is most often involved, the localised lesion appearing as a firm, annular thickening of the intestinal wall by a greyish-white homogeneous tissue, which may almost completely occlude the bowel lumen (***259***). The mesenteric lymph nodes, and especially those near the ileo-caeco-colic junction, are grossly enlarged and have a cut surface similar to that of the lymph nodes in the multicentric type. In some cases the intestinal lesion is small, the main feature being a group of very enlarged mesenteric nodes.

A common variant, seen mainly in the cat, is when the renal cortices are bilaterally infiltrated by masses of lymphosarcomatous tissue, leading to progressive renal failure

(***260***). The liver may be similarly involved, being grossly enlarged and having a very accentuated lobular pattern due to infiltration of the portal tracts by neoplastic cells (***261***).

Thymic lymphosarcomas tend to occur in younger animals, usually under three years of age. Affected animals often die with little warning, perhaps after a short illness characterised by inappetence and respiratory distress. A large radio-opaque mass occupying the anterior half of the thorax is visible on radiography (***262** and **263***) and thoracic fluid aspirates contain masses of abnormal lymphoblastic cells (***264***).

Most cases in horses are alimentary in type (***265***) with loss of condition accompanied by diarrhoea being the most frequent clinical signs.

Lymphadenopathy and skin tumours have also been described.

Haematology and histology

The anaemia is probably due to depressed erythropoiesis and increased haemolysis. Neutrophilia is frequently present, especially in advanced cases where tumour necrosis and secondary infection occur. Malignant circulating cells are not uncommon but frankly leukaemic cases are unusual.

Impression smears of lymph nodes can be of value in classification into histiocytic, lymphocytic and plasmacytic types.

The most characteristic change seen in the lymph nodes is a complete loss of the normal architecture which is replaced by a homogeneous sheet of closely packed lymphoid cells, including large and small lymphocytes as well as lymphoblastic types (***266***). The nucleus is round or ovoid and mitotic figures are variable in frequency. Vacuolated histiocytes occur in some tumours giving a so-called 'starry sky' appearance.

Aetiology

The disease in the cat is transmissible and is caused by an oncorna virus (***267***). In affected cats smears of peripheral blood or bone marrow treated with fluorescein conjugated rabbit anti-feline leukaemia virus serum show bright green fluorescence which is diagnostic for the presence of virus (***268***). This is also a useful screening test for cats which have not developed the clinical disease.

C type particles similar to those described in the cat have also been seen in the dog, but a causal relationship has not been established.

Treatment and prognosis

In the cat the clinical course of the disease is short, most cases being dead within eight weeks of diagnosis. In the alimentary form in all species euthanasia is usually carried out soon after diagnosis. Most cases of multicentric disease in the dog are dead within three months of the first consultation.

Following cortico-steroid therapy in the dog (*2.5mg/kg bodyweight prednisolone or 0.02mg/kg bodyweight betamethasone daily*) there is usually improvement in appetite and well-being, and some lymph node regression, although there is no evidence that life is prolonged. Other drugs which have been used include azathioprine (*2–5mg/kg*), chlorambucil (*0.2–0.3mg/kg*), cyclophosphamide (*0.3–1mg/kg*) and L-asparaginase (*1,000–2,500 units intravenously*). In Veterinary Schools combinations of drugs have been used with some limited success, e.g. the simultaneous administration of vinblastine, cytosine arabinoside, cyclophosphamide, prednisolone and l-asparaginase.

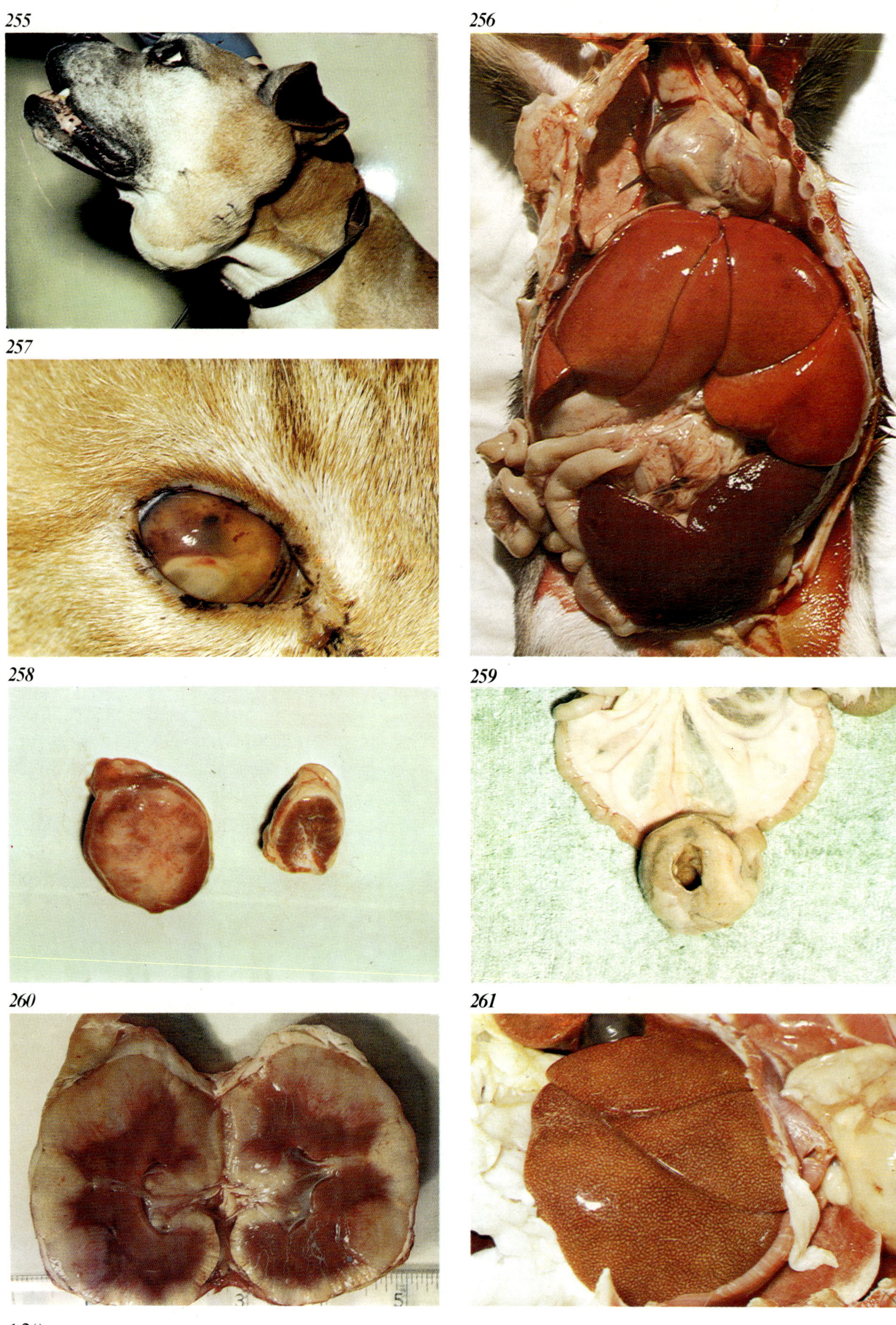
255
256
257
258
259
260
261

255 *Gross enlargement of the parotid and submandibular lymph nodes in canine multicentric lymphosarcoma.*

256 *Hepatosplenomegaly in canine lymphosarcoma.*

257 *Infiltration of the anterior chamber of the eye by lymphocytes in feline lymphosarcoma. When the animal is standing the cells sediment into the angle of filtration.*

258 *Cut surface of a lymphosarcomatous lymph node. Note the loss of internal architecture and the bulging, oedematous appearance. The node on the right is hyperplastic.*

259 *Solitary lymphosarcomatous nodule in the wall of the small intestine – cat.*

260 *Diffuse infiltration of the renal cortex by lymphosarcomatous tissue – cat. This lesion is nearly always bilateral.*

261 *Selective infiltration of the portal tracts by lymphosarcoma cells causing accentuation of the normal lobular pattern – cat.*

262 *Radiographic appearance of thymic lymphosarcoma – dog.*

Leukaemia

Leukaemia is uncommon in the dog and cat and very rare in the horse although some cases of lymphosarcoma in the dog and cat have a leukaemic blood picture and could be classified as lymphocytic leukaemia. Cases of true lymphocytic leukaemia in the dog show only an enlarged liver and spleen, with large numbers (*up to 500,000mm*^{3}) of circulating lymphocytes and lymphoblasts (***269***). Skin lesions may develop (***270***) and clinical signs attributable to meningeal infiltration may occur.

262

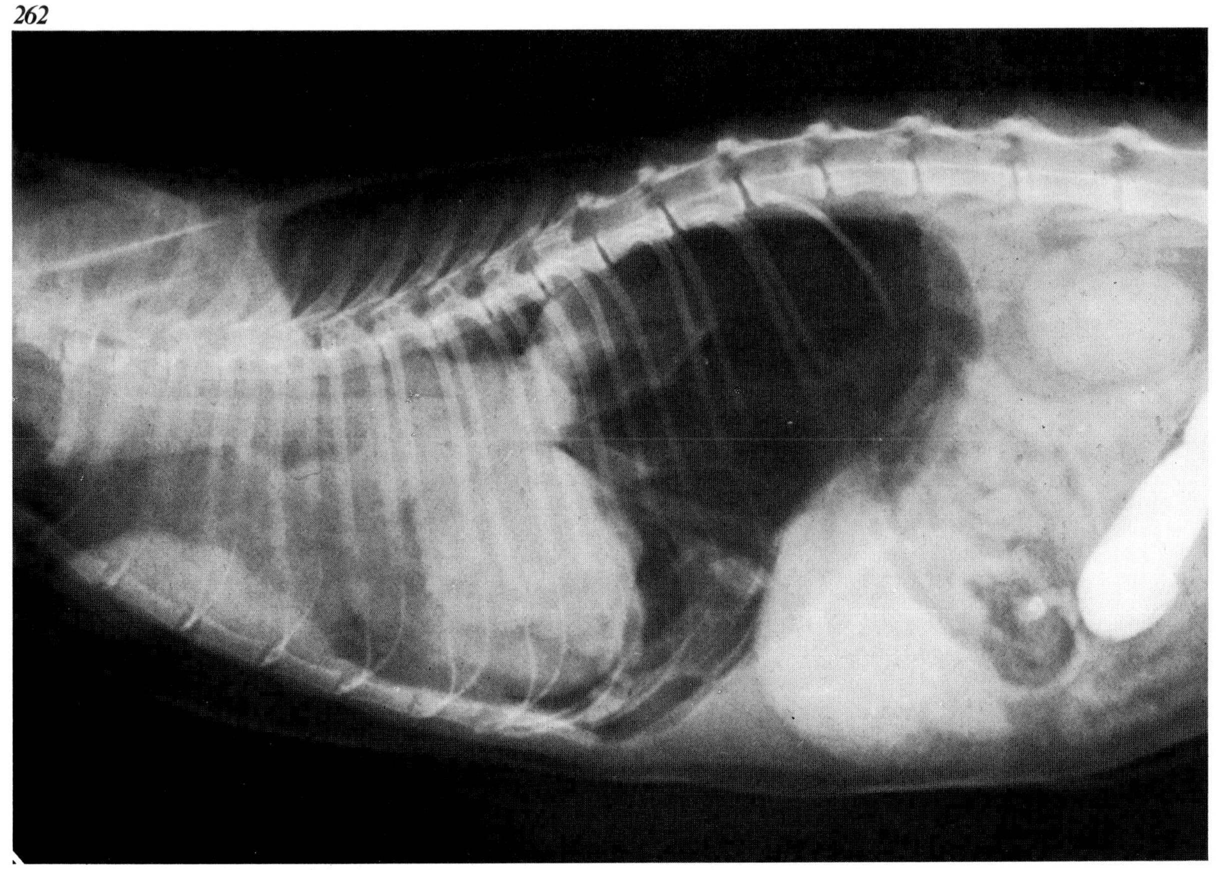

263 *Thymic lymphosarcoma occupying most of the anterior part of the chest – dog. These tumours are often encapsulated and confined to the thymic areas.*

264 *Smear of thoracic exudate from a dog with thymic lymphosarcoma. Giemsa stain.*

265 *Diffuse alimentary lymphosarcoma in the small intestine of a 10-year-old mare. The entire length of the intestine was involved. Note the enormously enlarged lymphoid follicles with ulceration of the overlying mucosa.*

266 *Lymphosarcoma – dog. The cells are closely packed, not arranged in any pattern and have a central nucleus with a narrow rim of cytoplasm. H & E.*

267 *Electron micrograph of oncornavirus (C type) particle, budding from the surface of a transformed cell – cat.*

268 *Apple green fluorescence of transformed lymphoblasts containing oncornavirus – cat.*

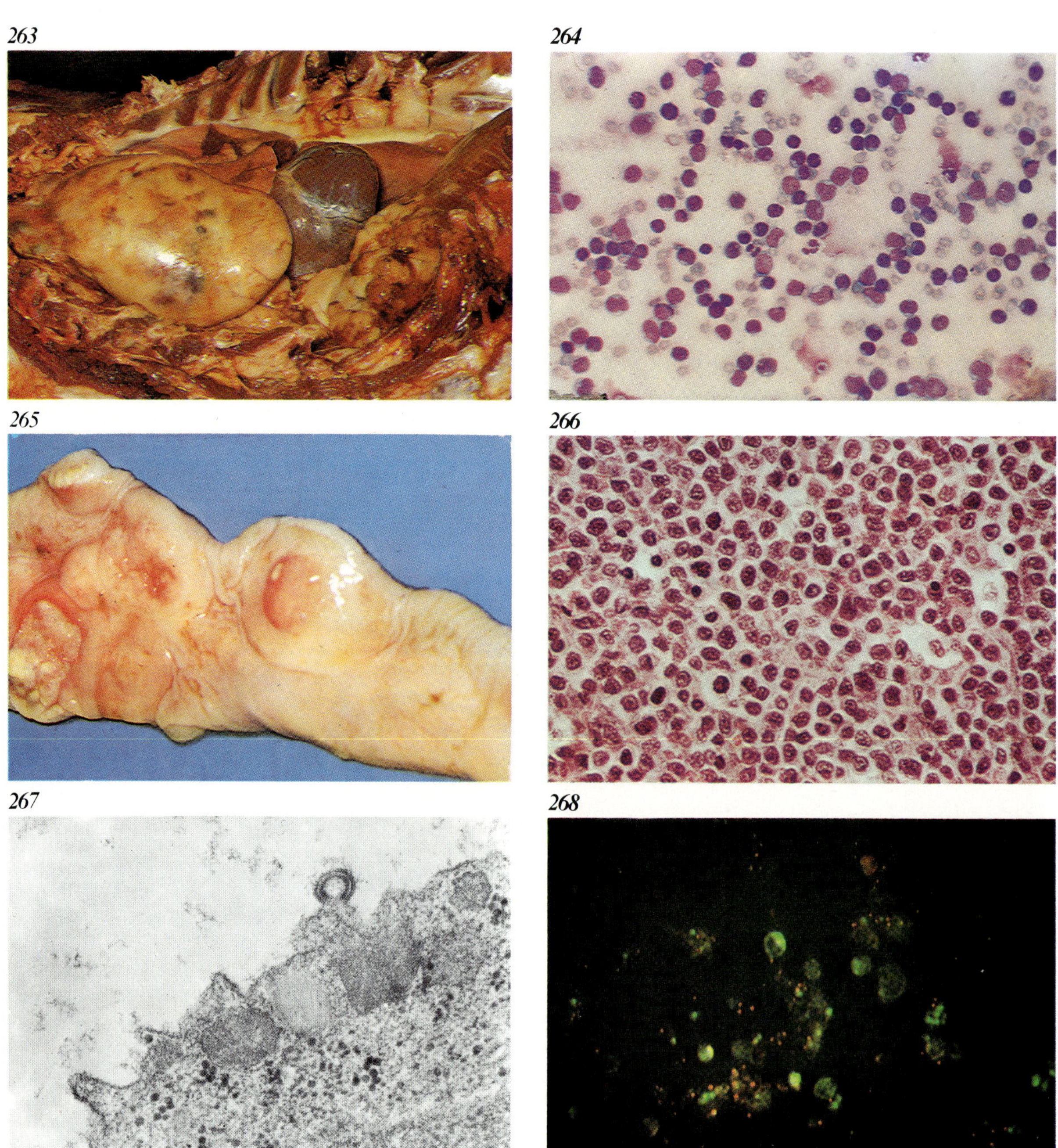

269 *Buffy coat of dog with leukaemia. The total white cell count was 200,000/mm^3, 99% of which were lymphoblasts.*

270 *Infiltration of the skin by malignant lymphoblasts in a dog with leukaemia.*

271 *Malignant haemangioendothelioma of the wall of the right atrium – dog.*

272 *Malignant haemangioendothelioma of the canine spleen.*

273 *Multiple hepatic metastases from a splenic haemangioendothelioma – dog.*

274 *Splenic haematoma – dog.*

269

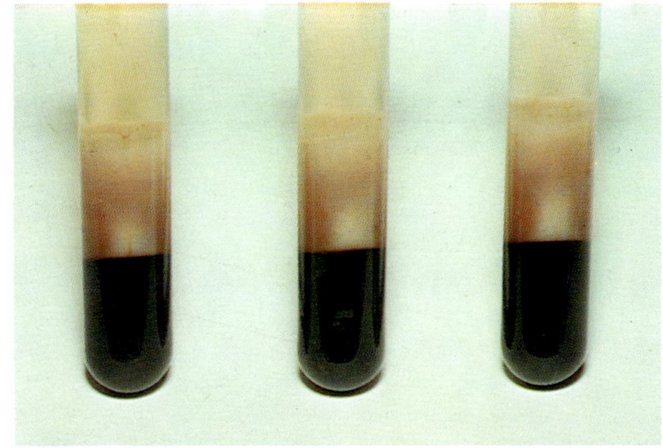

270

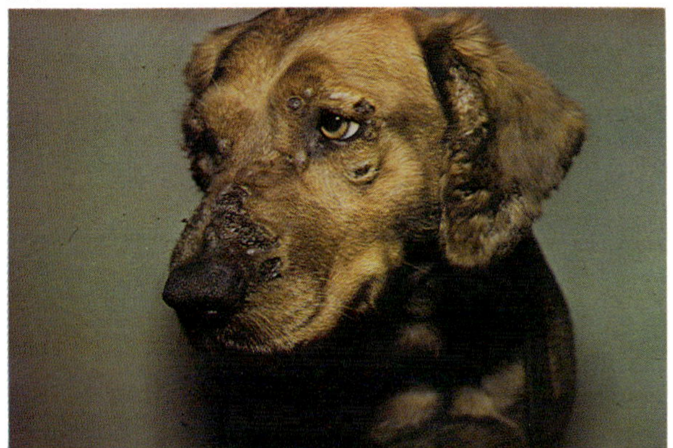

271

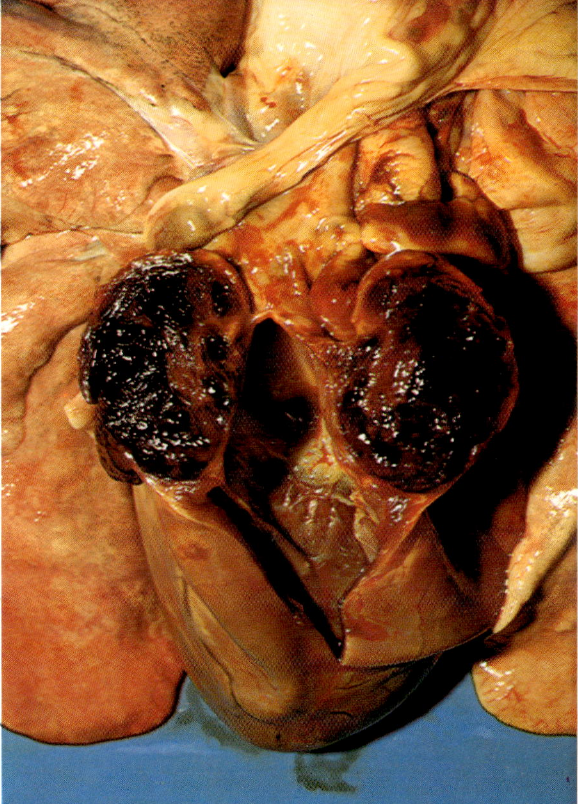

272

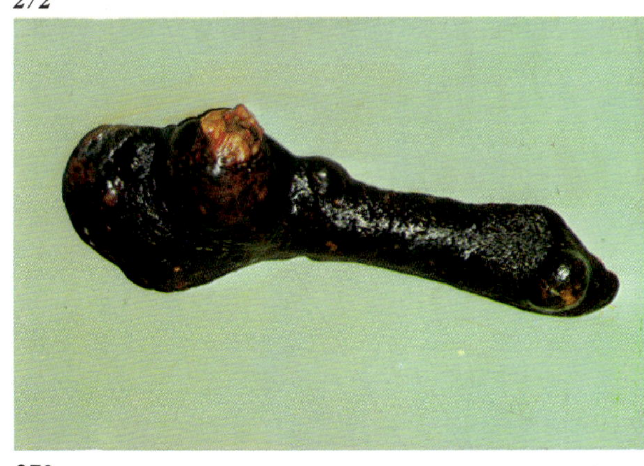

273

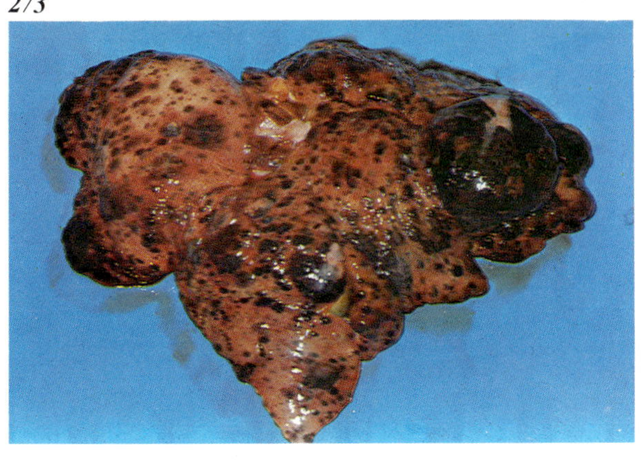

274

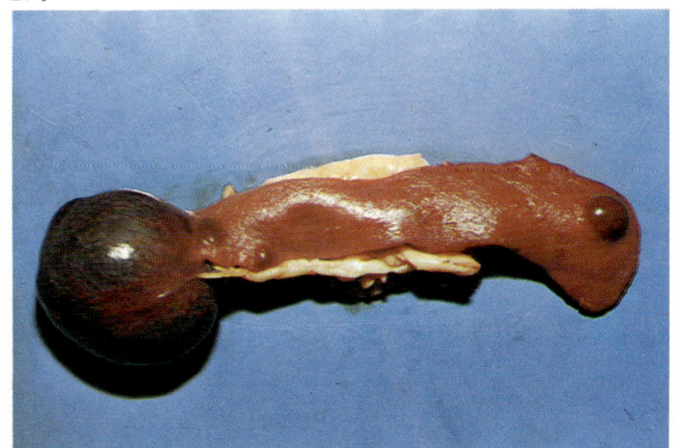

Myelogenous leukaemia is rare. It arises from the myeloid cells of the bone marrow and circulating white cell counts can be very high, with large numbers of 'blast' forms present. The bone marrow is white or greyish-red and there is usually enlargement of liver and spleen. Animals are usually severely anaemic and seldom live long following diagnosis. Monocytic leukaemia has been described in the cat.

Plasma Cell Myelomas

Tumours usually develop in bone (*see page 102*) but occasionally may develop in spleen, skin, or other solid viscera.

TUMOURS OF THE VASCULAR ENDOTHELIUM

Malignant Haemangioendotheliomas

Malignant haemangioendothelioma of the skin is described on page 38. Primary tumours of this type are also seen arising from the myocardium, especially of the right atrium (*271*), and the spleen (*272*). These tumours are highly malignant and widespread metastasis to the liver (*273*) and lungs is common. Sudden death may occur due to rupture of the tumour, followed by massive haemorrhage.

Cavernous Haemangiomas

Cavernous haemangioma of the skin is described on page 38. The spleen is frequently involved in dogs, and the spleen or liver in horses. In the dog it is often possible to remove the affected spleen surgically, following which the prognosis is favourable.

NON-NEOPLASTIC TUMOUR-LIKE LESIONS

Splenic Haematomas

Non-neoplastic haematomas of the spleen are frequently confused with tumours in dogs. They appear as very large, spherical, rather spongy masses (*274*) with a dark red, gelatinous cut surface. Histologically they are composed of sheets of degenerating red cells or fibrin surrounded by a thick fibrous capsule. Following surgical excision of the spleen the prognosis in these cases is good.

Chapter 12
The Respiratory System

Primary tumours of the respiratory tract in animals are relatively uncommon but may arise from the tissues of either the nasal chambers or the lungs themselves. Benign tumours include nasal polyps and adenomas derived from the nasal mucosa. Malignant tumours, which are more common, include carcinomas and osteosarcomas in the nasal chambers and carcinomas of the lung.

A rather unusual lesion, seen only in the horse, is the 'progressive haematoma of the ethmoid region' which may not be a true neoplasm.

The lungs are a common site for the development of metastatic tumours in all species.

TUMOURS OF THE UPPER RESPIRATORY TRACT

Nasal Polyps

Occurrence and gross appearance

Polyps arise from the nasal mucosa and are seen most often in horses. They are usually unilateral, smooth, pedunculated, firm and rubbery, and may ulcerate, bleed, or become secondarily infected. They sometimes appear at the nostril, when diagnosis is straightforward but most cases require more detailed examination. Clinical signs include sneezing, respiratory distress, and haemorrhage from the nostril.

Histological appearance

Polyps are composed of dense fibrous tissue and resemble fibromas, although whorls of cells are not seen. Polyps which contain spicules of cancellous bone have also been described. They are covered by a cuboidal or columnar epithelium which is frequently eroded and infiltrated by inflammatory cells.

Aetiology

Chronic inflammation may play a part in the aetiology of some polyps.

Treatment and prognosis

Most polyps cannot be removed via the nostril and it is usually necessary to trephine, taking care not to injure the nasal septum. Haemorrhage may be profuse, but following skilled surgical excision, recurrence is rare.

Nasal Carcinomas

Occurrence and gross appearance

Adenocarcinomas arising from the columnar epithelium of the nasal chamber and the sinuses occur in all three species and have also been described in the guttural pouch in horses. Although they are usually unilateral, the affected side is extensively involved, with almost total destruction of the turbinate bones. The nasal chamber, and sometimes the frontal sinus, becomes blocked by a pale, brownish-grey, friable tissue (***275***) giving rise to the clinical signs of 'snoring' respiration, unilateral mucopurulent nasal discharge and dullness on percussion. In many cases the tumour causes obvious distortion of the maxilla or frontal bone, sometimes with displacement of the eye. Dorso-ventral radiographs reveal the presence of a diffuse, radio-opaque material in the affected chamber, with evidence of erosion of the overlying bone (***276***).

Squamous cell carcinomas are usually confined to the region of the external nares, where they are firm, pale, and very erosive.

Histological appearance

Most tumours are very poorly differentiated and are composed of a closely packed, homogeneous sheet of large, hyperchromatic cells not arranged in any definite architectural pattern (***277***). In some cases, however, acini composed of large epithelial cells are seen (***278***).

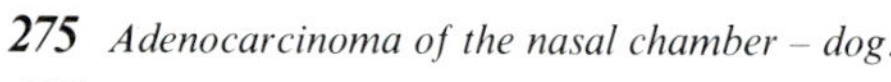

275 *Adenocarcinoma of the nasal chamber – dog.*

275

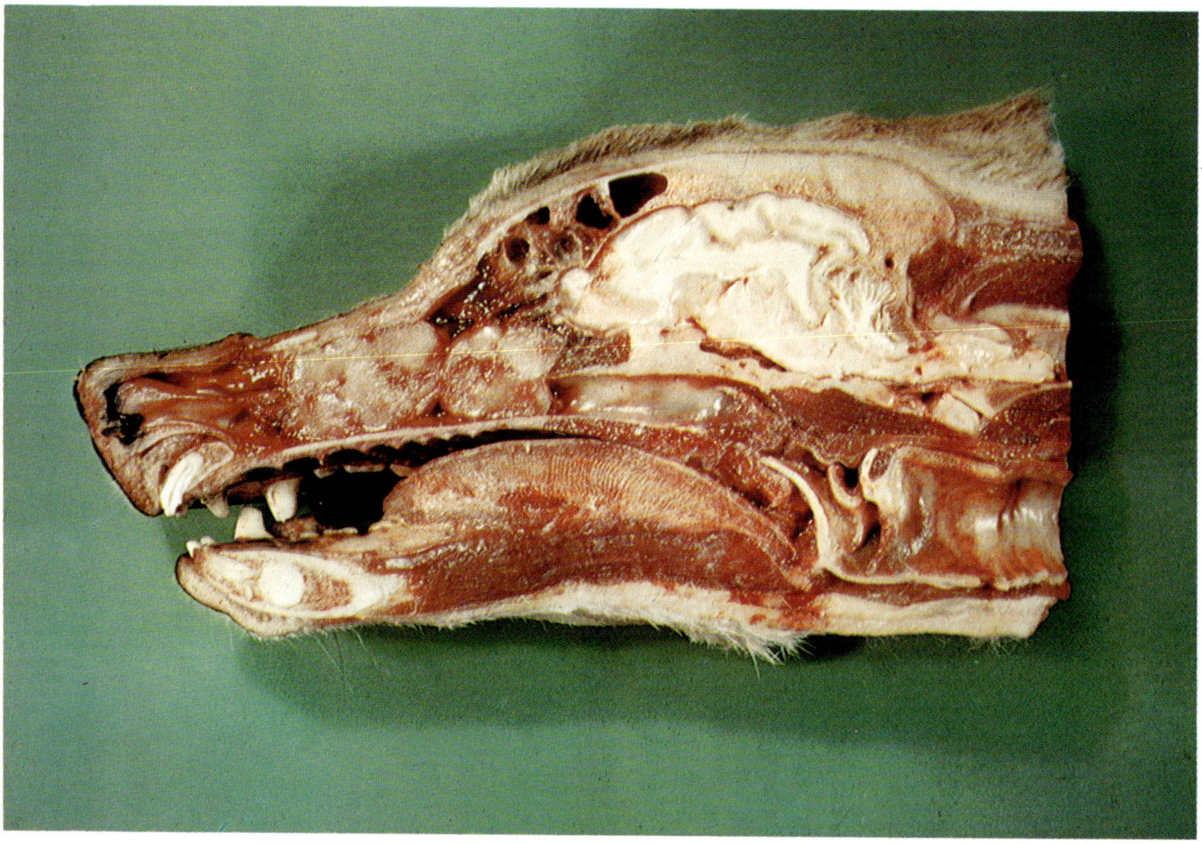

276 *Radiographic appearance of a nasal adenocarcinoma in the left nasal chamber of a dog. Note the extensive destruction of the overlying bone.*

276

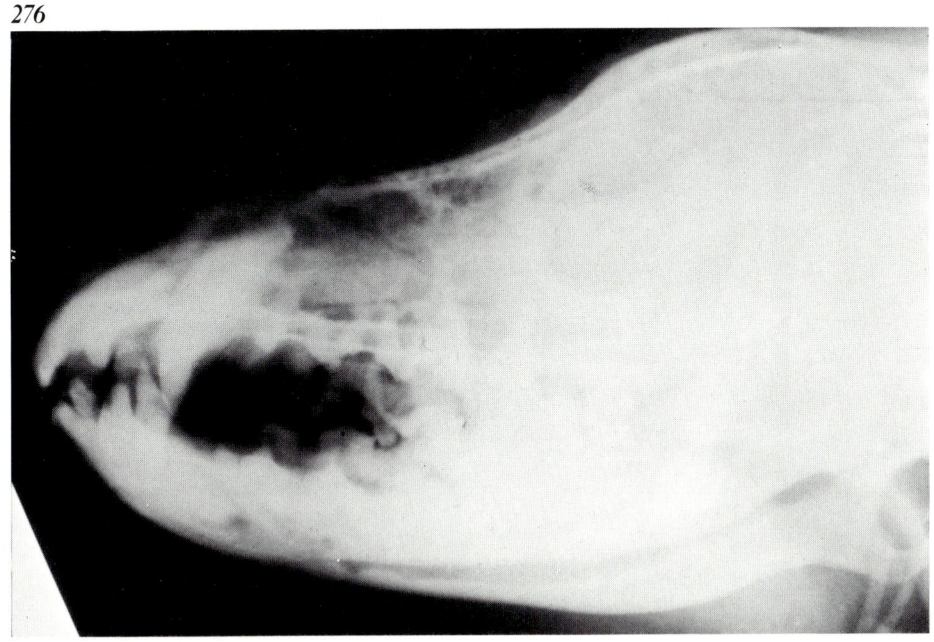

277 *Poorly differentiated adenocarcinoma of the nasal chamber – dog. H & E.*

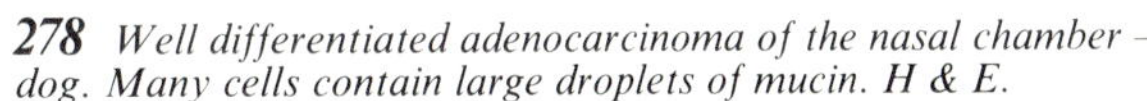

278 *Well differentiated adenocarcinoma of the nasal chamber – dog. Many cells contain large droplets of mucin. H & E.*

277

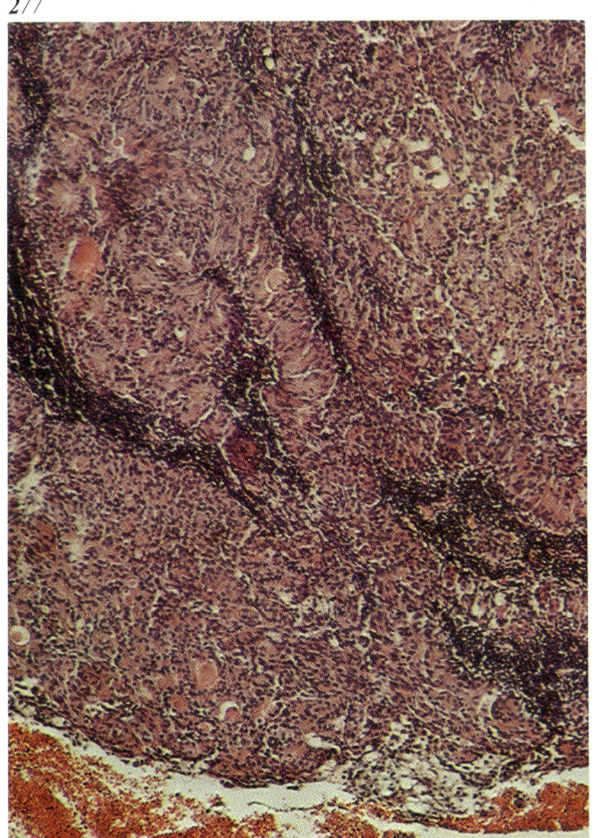

278

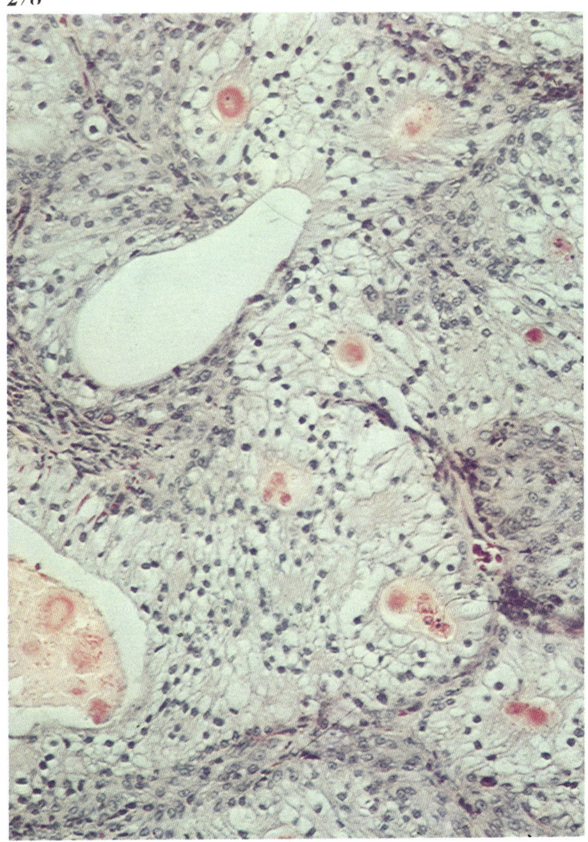

Aetiology

Unknown. An enzootic form of carcinoma of the ethmo-turbinates has occurred in horses in Sweden.

Treatment and prognosis

The prognosis is always poor. In the dog and cat very extensive and radical surgery is necessary to effect a cure and many cases are too advanced for this treatment when first seen. Radiotherapy alone is only a palliative measure but a combination of X-irradiation and surgery is worth consideration. Metastasis is very unusual from tumours in this site even though they appear poorly differentiated histologically.

Progressive Haematomas of the Ethmoid Region in the Horse (Ethmoidal Giant Cell Tumours)

Occurrence and gross appearance

This condition has been described only in horses. Clinical manifestations include haemorrhagic or mucopurulent nasal discharge, and, eventually, 'snoring' respirations. Diagnosis may be made by radiography (*279*) and endoscopy. The lesion usually appears

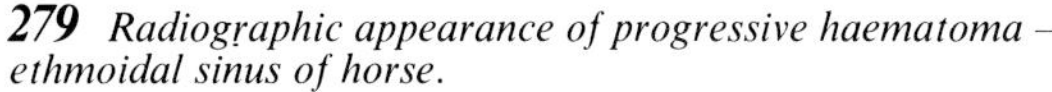

279 *Radiographic appearance of progressive haematoma – ethmoidal sinus of horse.*

279

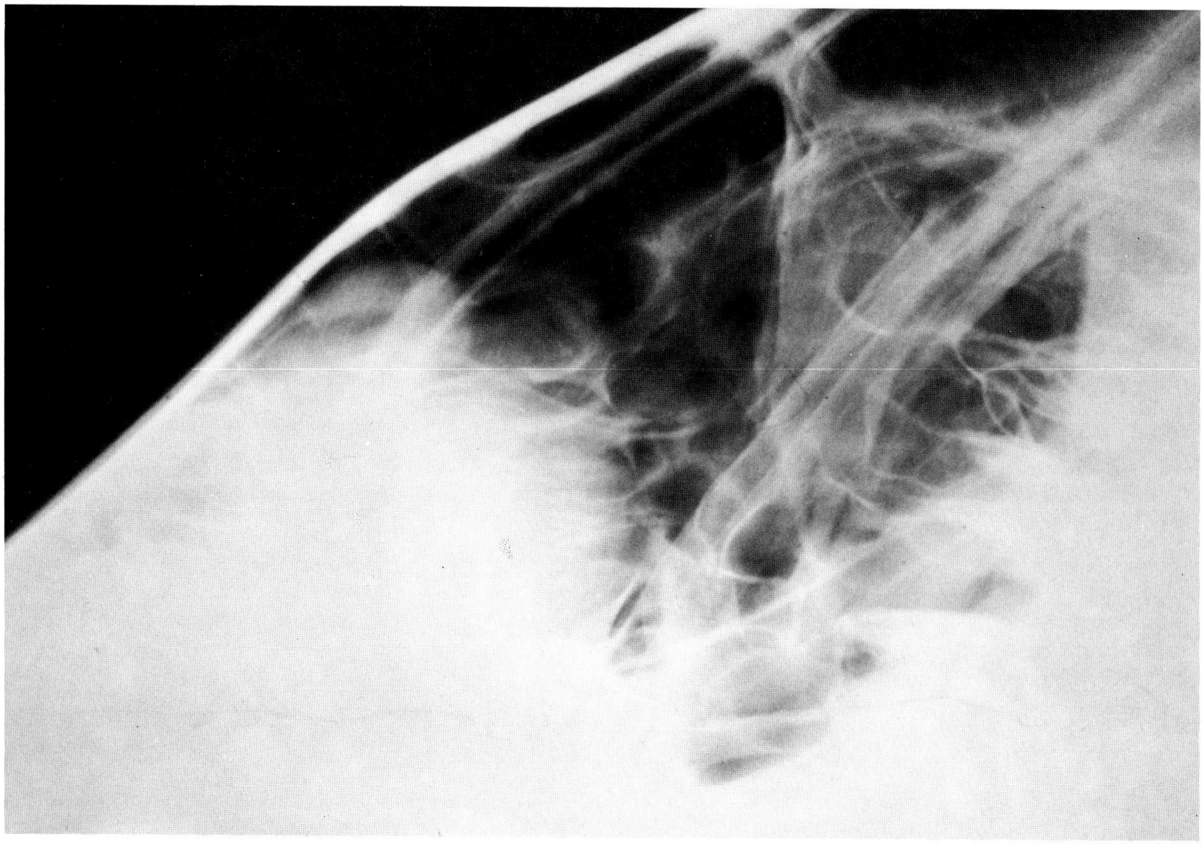

grossly as a unilateral, though occasionally bilateral, firm, ulcerated mass in the posterior aspect of the nasal cavity, apparently arising from the ethmoidal meatus in the region of the ethmoid labyrinth and extending for a variable distance into the nasal cavity (***280***), or nasopharynx. The cut surface is dark reddish-brown in colour, extensively mottled by haemorrhage and may be surrounded by a thick fibrous capsule. Similar, although smaller, lesions may arise from other sites in the paranasal sinuses.

Histological appearance

The most striking feature of these lesions is their pleomorphism. The central zone generally consists of both old and more recent haemorrhage, surrounded by a dense fibrous stroma containing numerous macrophages, the cytoplasm of which is packed with haemosiderin. In some areas however the most obvious feature is the presence of many, irregularly shaped, multinucleate giant cells (***281***). Giant cells are not distributed evenly throughout the mass but tend to occur in densely packed foci. There is usually evidence of pressure necrosis of the surrounding bone.

Aetiology

There is still considerable confusion as to the underlying nature of this lesion and to whether or not it is truly neoplastic. Some workers believe that it is not a true tumour but a result of chronic infection or repeated haemorrhage, and the pleomorphic histological appearance is certainly more suggestive of this.

Treatment and prognosis

Excision of the entire mass and ethmoid labyrinth is possible following a surgical approach through the frontal and maxillary sinus. Haemorrhage is severe.

Following excision, local recurrence is seen in more than 30% of cases and sometimes a similar lesion develops on the opposite side. The prognosis should thus be guarded.

TUMOURS OF THE LUNG

Adenomas and Carcinomas

Occurrence and gross appearance

Adenomas and carcinomas of the lung are rare in the horse and uncommon in the dog and cat. In one survey in the USA primary lung cancers in the dog occurred at a rate of 0.6% of all canine necropsies. Most tumours are found in old dogs and cats, with adenomas tending to be large, pale, solitary, roughly spherical nodules (***282***), which may replace an entire lobe, whilst carcinomas are usually multiple due to the presence of extensive intra-pulmonary metastases (***283***). Before making a diagnosis of primary lung tumour, the possibility of a primary tumour elsewhere must be excluded.

Clinical signs are variable and include cough, abdominal breathing, cyanosis, anorexia and weight loss.

Radiographs show large opaque masses in one or more lobes of the lung and, more rarely, diffuse opacity over all lobes.

280

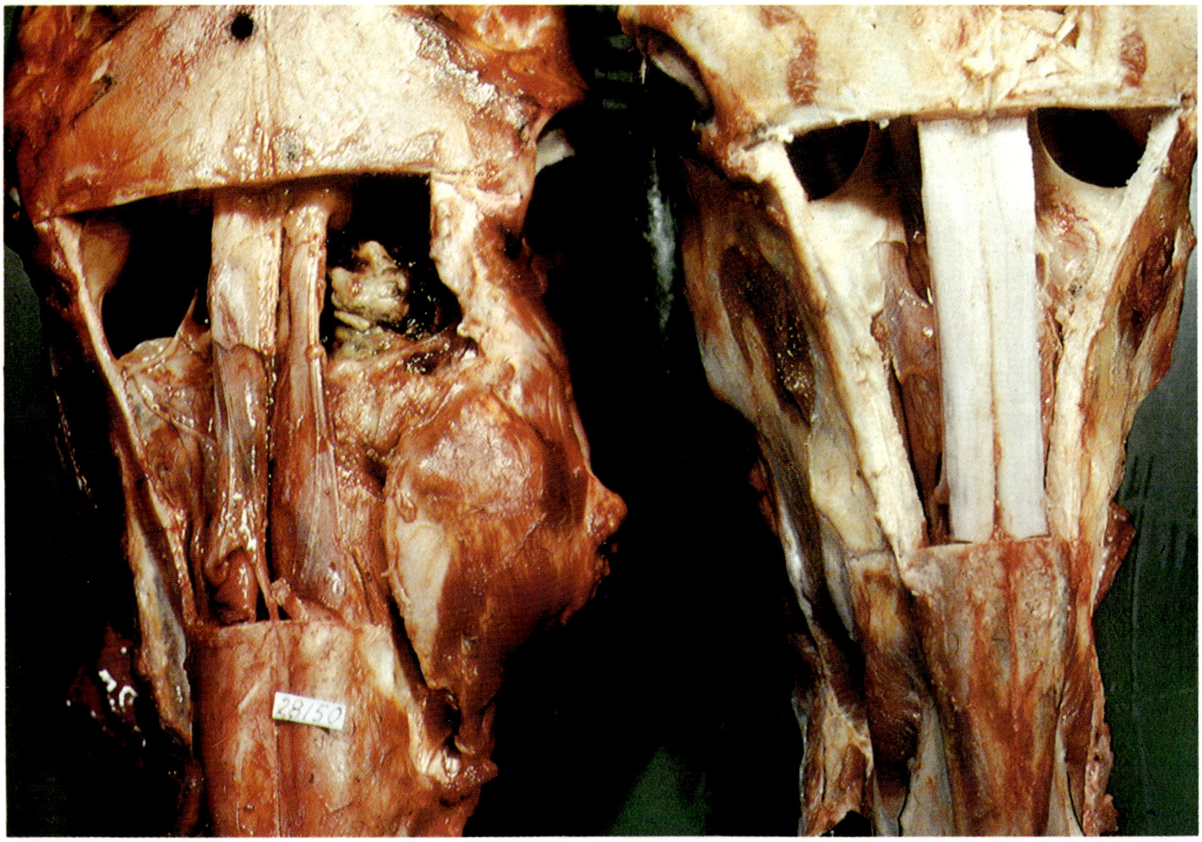

281

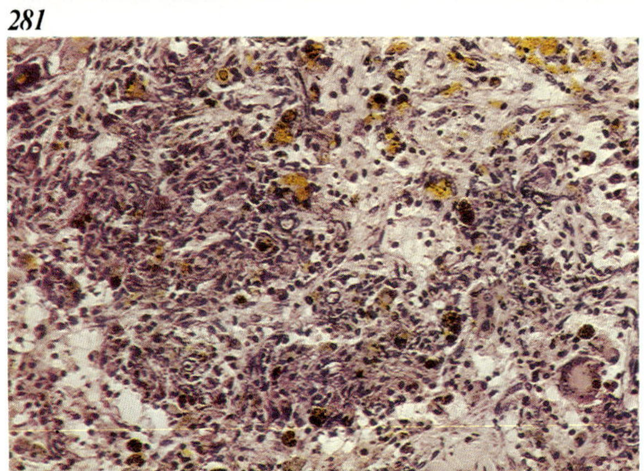

282

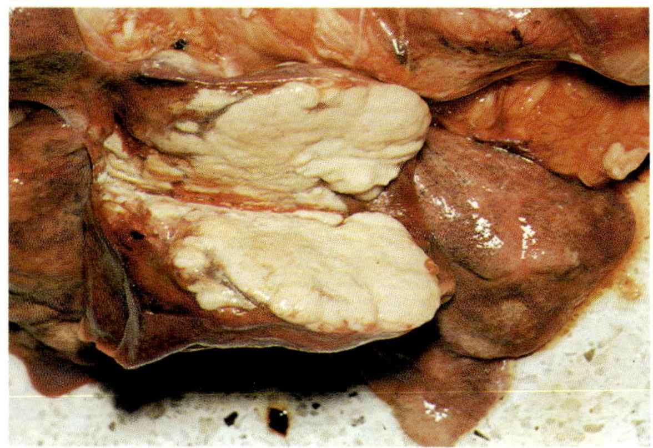

283

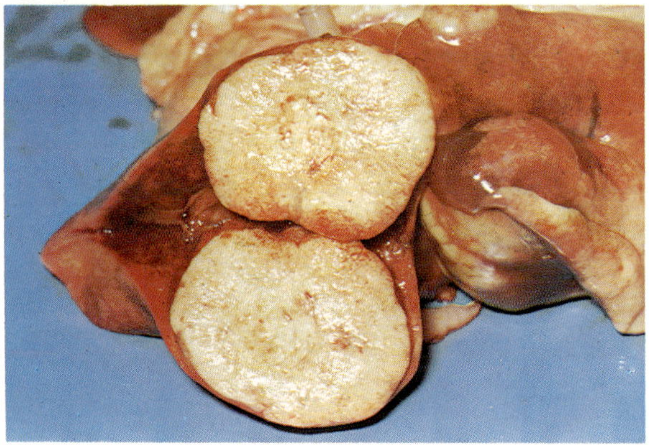

280 *Large progressive haematoma in the left nasal chamber – horse. The surrounding bone has been distorted by the mass. The skull on the right is normal and has been included for comparison.*

281 *Multinucleate giant cells and syncytia of macrophages in progressive ethmoid haematoma. H & E.*

282 *Cut surface of pulmonary adenoma in a six-year-old Boxer bitch.*

283 *Multiple secondaries from pulmonary adenocarcinoma – dog. Note the similarity between the appearance of these malignant tumours and the benign tumours in **282**.*

Histological appearance

In the dog adenocarcinomas are of two types – columnar cell or bronchogenic carcinoma (***284***), and the cuboidal cell or bronchiolar alveolar type (***285***). Rarely, primary squamous cell carcinomas occur and have a similar appearance to those in other sites. In cats most carcinomas are of the columnar cell type, although many are anaplastic and may show a tendency towards keratinisation.

It is usually very difficult to distinguish benign from malignant tumours on histological criteria alone, apparently circumscribed and well differentiated lesions sometimes giving rise to widespread secondaries following lobectomy.

284 *Columnar cell adenocarcinoma of lung – cat. H & E.*

284

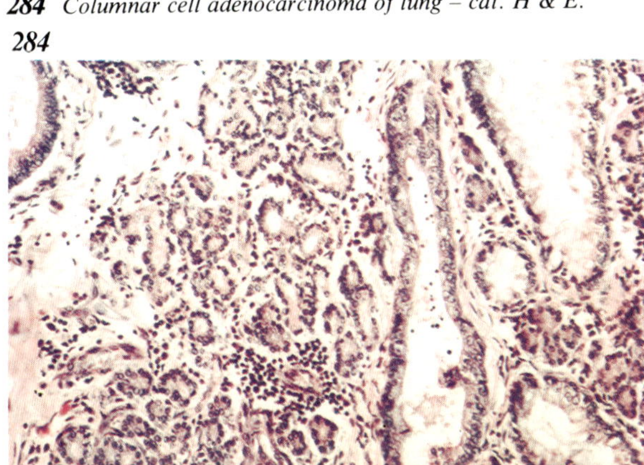

285 *Cuboidal cell adenocarcinoma of lung – dog. H & E.*

285

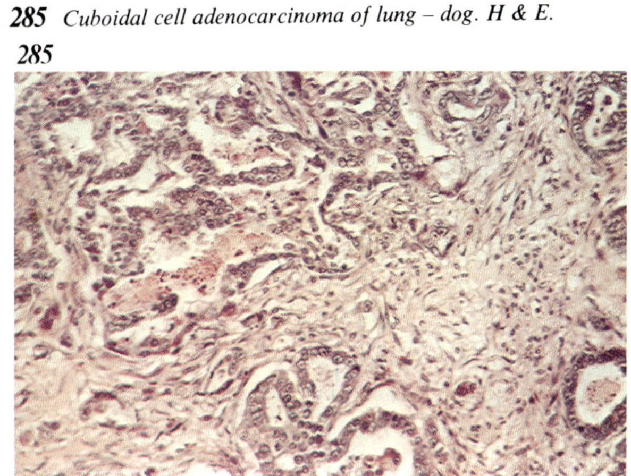

Treatment and prognosis

The prognosis should always be guarded because of the frequency of intra-pulmonary metastasis, although lobectomy has proved successful in the treatment of solitary adenomas in a few dogs.

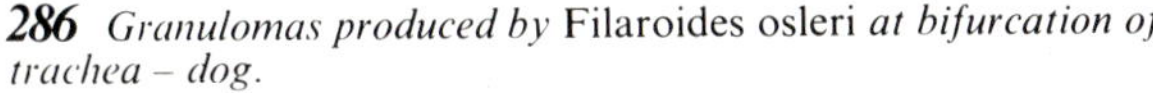

286 *Granulomas produced by* Filaroides osleri *at bifurcation of trachea – dog.*

286

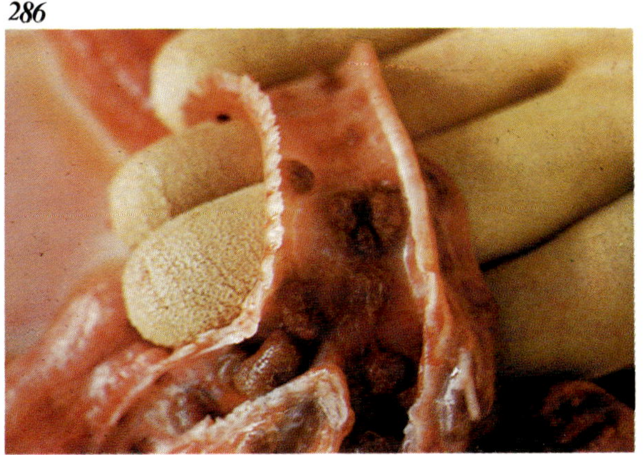

287 *Masses of embryonated eggs of* Aelurostrongylus abstrusus *in cat lung. Note the granulomatous inflammatory reaction which is elicited by the parasite.*

287

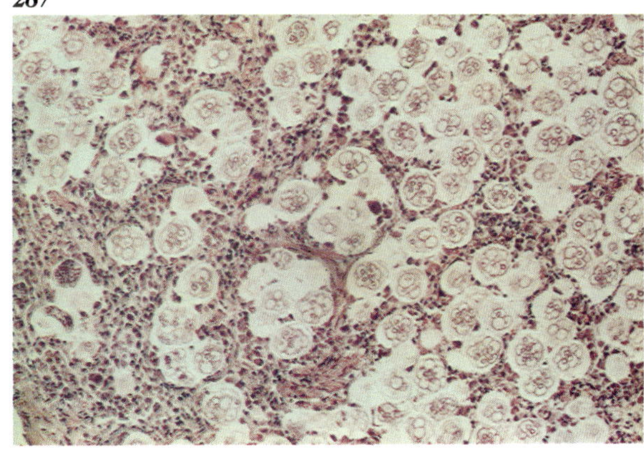

NON-NEOPLASTIC TUMOUR-LIKE LESIONS

Granulomas

There are a number of diseases which produce granulomas in the respiratory tract, the lesions sometimes being confused with neoplasms, and of these the parasitic granulomas produced by *Filaroides osleri* in the canine trachea and bronchi, and *Aelurostrongylus abstrusus* in the feline lung, are the most important.

The most common clinical sign of Filaroides infestation is chronic coughing, and bronchoscopy reveals the presence of multiple firm, raised nodules, 1–2cm in diameter at the bifurcation of the trachea (***286***), within which the parasites can sometimes be seen.

Lesions in the lung caused by *Aelurostrongylus* are very difficult to distinguish from lung secondaries on gross examination. They occur mainly in the diaphragmatic lobes, and appear as multiple small, roughly spherical greyish nodules, a few millimetres in diameter, scattered throughout the lung parenchyma. Histologically, the appearance is of a granulomatous inflammatory reaction mainly around masses of eggs and larvae (***287***). Another very conspicuous feature is the marked hypertrophy of the smooth muscle in the walls of the pulmonary arterioles.

Chapter 13
The Eye

Intra-ocular tumours are uncommon. The commonest single type is the melanoma, although adenomas, adenocarcinomas and medullo-epitheliomas arising from the ciliary bodies also occur and lymphosarcomas or leukaemia in the dog and cat can be manifested as eye lesions (*see page 129*).

Intra-ocular metastases from oral melanomas and transmissible venereal tumours have been described.

Intra-ocular Melanomas

Occurrence and gross appearance

Melanomas are seen most often in dogs and rarely in cats. They are usually unilateral and appear as a very darkly pigmented mass arising from the iris or ciliary body. They may push the iris forward and cause it to adhere to the cornea. They are variable in size, usually measuring from 0.5–2cm in diameter, have an indistinct boundary and a black, homogeneous cut surface (***288***).

Histological appearance

Tumours are usually very well differentiated and composed of a closely packed sheet of polygonal cells, the normal architecture of which has been completely obscured by masses of melanin pigment (***289***). Occasionally less well differentiated, almost unpigmented tumours are seen.

Treatment and prognosis

The only form of treatment is enucleation of the globe, following which a complete cure is to be expected. Extra globular growth and metastasis is very unusual in animals.

Adenomas and Adenocarcinomas of the Ciliary Body

These are rare tumours which occur in all three species and which arise from the ciliary body epithelium. Differentiation between benign and malignant types is difficult and depends upon histological criteria since both tend to be small nodular lesions usually less than 1cm in diameter, roughly spherical and fairly well encapsulated. Clinical signs include glaucoma and blindness. The tumour may become visible through the cornea (***290***) and produce an anterior synechia. The cut surface of the tumour is characteristically white, firm, and homogeneous (***291***), although small areas of pigmentation are sometimes apparent.

Histological appearance

Adenomas consist of a loose connective tissue stroma which contains closely packed, cuboidal cells which are arranged as irregular acini chains, or papillary structures.

Carcinomas have a very similar appearance but the cells tend to be smaller and more hyperchromatic (*292*).

Treatment and prognosis

The treatment of choice is enucleation of the globe and as these tumours do not metastasise the prognosis following this procedure is good.

288 *Melanoma of the iris – dog.*

289 *Melanoma of the ciliary body. These tumours are generally well differentiated and so heavily pigmented that the structure of the cells is completely obscured. H & E.*

290 *Adenocarcinoma of the ciliary body – dog.*

291 *Cut surface of ciliary body adenocarcinoma – dog.*

292 *Ciliary body adenocarcinoma. The cells are hyperchromatic and are forming irregular, branching papillae. H & E.*

288

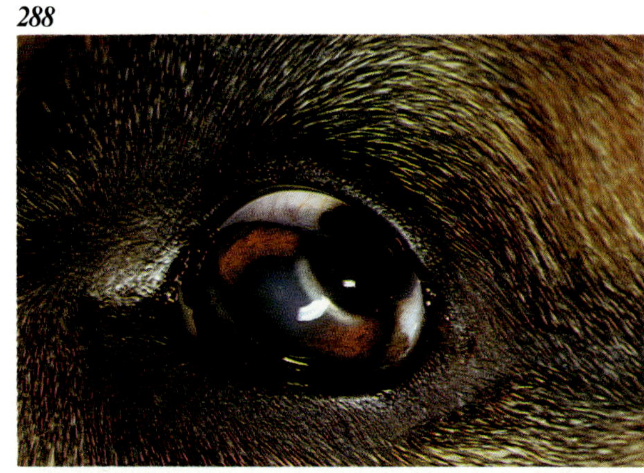

289

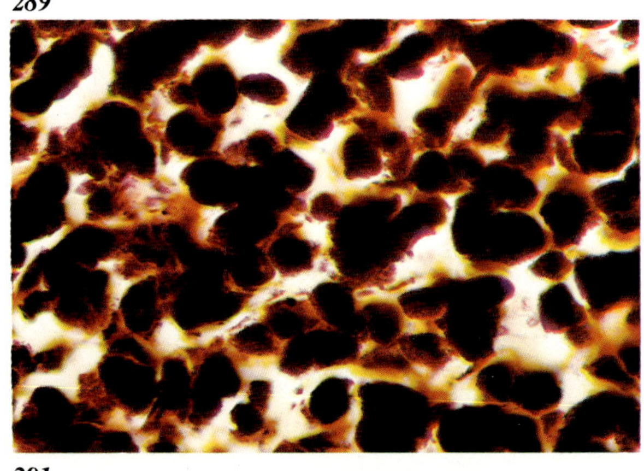

290

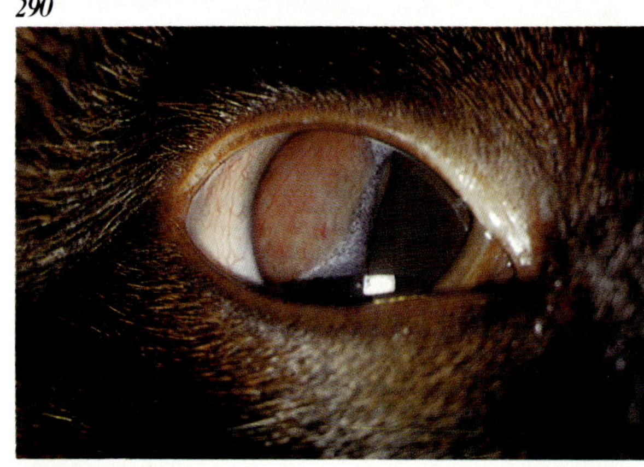

291

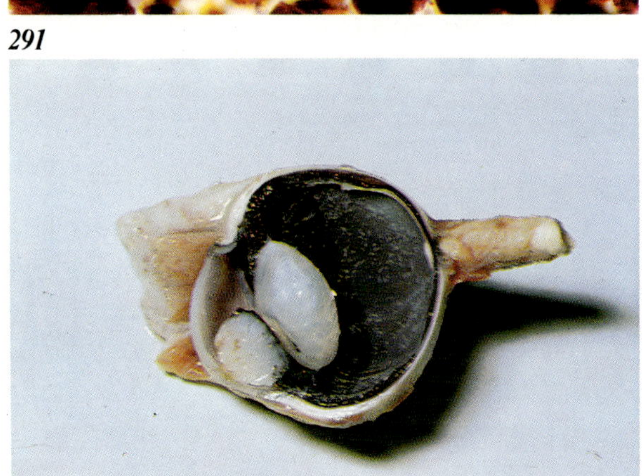

292

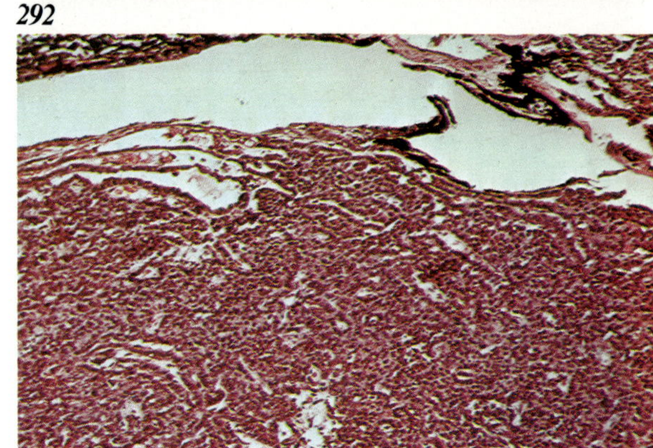

INDEX

(The references printed in italic type are to page numbers and those in **bold** *are to picture and caption numbers.)*